CONTENTS

vii **Foreword**
Dr. Zaven Khachaturian, Director
Ronald and Nancy Reagan Center
for Alzheimer's Research

1 **What Alzheimer's Disease Is**

7 **What Alzheimer's Disease Is Not**

17 **Who Is at Risk for Alzheimer's Disease**

31 **What Happens to the Patient
with Alzheimer's Disease**

39 **What Happens to the Brain
with Alzheimer's Disease**

63 **Acetylcholine**

71 **Aluminum**

77 **Heredity and Alzheimer's Disease**

89 **Apolipoprotein E and the
Susceptibility Genes**

99 **Amyloid ß Peptide**

107 **Neurofibrillary Tangles**

113 **Inflammation**

125 **New Directions**

137 **Green Barley Juice, Snake Oil,
and other Dubious Remedies**

145 **What You Can Do to Fight
Alzheimer's Disease**

155 **Reading List**

157 **Afterword**

159 **Acknowledgemen**

Foreword

ALTHOUGH ALZHEIMER'S DISEASE WAS FIRST described as a clinical entity in 1907, it has been always been part of the human condition. The Ancients were rarely confronted with it because for most of human history very few people survived beyond the age of 40 years. For those who did, the development of memory problems was assumed to be due to a rare consequence of aging. The term senility therefore came increasingly to signify not only the condition of being old, but also, by extension, the condition of being demented. The prospect of dementia with age seemed as incvitable as aging itself, with little hope of treatment or prevention.

This prevailing popular and scientific view of aging, dementia, and Alzheimer's disease did not change much until the late 1970's, when systematic studies began to capture the attention and the interest of the scientific community and the general public. Since then the number of articles and books on the general topics of aging, dementia, and Alzheimer's disease has steadily increased in both the scientific and lay media.

Scientists generally write for other scientists, leaving the difficult task of understanding complex biomedical research and translating it for the general public to journalists who may have little or no scientific background. As a result, important insights and critical information have sometimes been lost or misinterpreted. The present volume is one of the first to offer comprehensive coverage of Alzheimer's disease research, written for lay audiences by a working scientist.

Dr. Joseph Rogers has had extensive training and research experience at some of the world's leading laboratories and clinics. Since the beginning of his scientific career, which now spans more than two decades, he has been interested in understanding the aging brain and how it functions both in health and sickness. Although the recent history of Alzheimer's disease research in the United States is relatively brief, Dr. Rogers became involved in that history early in his career and very quickly began to make some of the most important and original contributions to this field of study. In particular, he was one of the first scientists to propose that the pathological conditions associated with Alzheimer's disease may reflect an inflammatory reaction in the brain. Some of his ideas have already proven to be promising leads for the development of treatments to delay the onset of symptoms.

Dr. Rogers' book, *Candle and Darkness*, is a valuable,

first-hand account of current research in Alzheimer's disease written by a well known scientist in the field. Most of all, however, it is a book that should be understandable to almost anyone, regardless of their scientific background, from the friends and family members of an Alzheimer's victim to established physicians with Alzheimer's patients. There are several excellent publications on the shelves that cover the care of Alzheimer's patients. To these, *Candle and Darkness* should be added as an essential companion volume for those who want to know more about the exciting new progress that is being made to understand, treat, and ultimately cure this increasingly pervasive human disorder.

Dr. Zaven Khachaturian
Director, Ronald and Nancy Reagan
Center for Alzheimer's Research

What Alzhiemer's Disease Is

IN 1906, DR. ALOIS ALZHEIMER, A GERMAN neurologist, looked into a microscope at autopsy tissue taken from the brain of one of his deceased patients. The patient had been demented. With a special silver stain that is still used today, what Dr. Alzheimer saw were microscopic lesions, now called senile or neuritic plaques, and nerve cells filled with tiny, black, thread-like filaments, now called neurofibrillary tangles. These plaques and tangles are the classic hallmarks of the disease that came to be named for the man who first noticed them. They are the stigmata of Alzheimer's disease.

Dr. Alzheimer wrote up his findings and presented them at a scientific meeting. No one paid much attention —the record shows that there were no questions or comments after the lecture. A few years later, however, one of Dr. Alzheimer's more famous colleagues examined brain samples from other patients who had died with similar symptoms of dementia. He also found profuse plaques, tangles, and nerve cell loss, results that were soon widely confirmed. Alzheimer's disease had been discovered.

Or had it? In fact, Alzheimer's has probably been with us for as long as people have lived long enough to get the disorder. We just called it something else: senility. This isn't satisfactory on several counts. First, as it is typically used, "senility" is a very imprecise term. Uncle Warren, who keeps repeating the same jokes to the same people every day, is said to be getting senile. Aunt Michelle, who can't seem to follow Uncle Warren's jokes anymore, has gotten senile. And Uncle Joe, who just jabbers a lot at the TV, is completely senile. Such vagueness is of little use in modern medicine. In fact, technically to say that someone is senile only means that he or she is in the senium, age sixty or more. For this reason, you should probably be careful about how you use the word: by a textbook definition you may soon be senile yourself, if you aren't already.

"Senile dementia," a term you may also hear a lot in the context of Alzheimer's disease, is more precise, but still inadequate. It means that a patient is old (in the senium) and demented (pathologically forgetful or cognitively impaired to the point where the patient can neither think straight nor function as an independent adult). Uncle Joe, Uncle Warren, and Aunt Michelle may all be in various stages of senility, but only Uncle Joe has senile dementia. Of the three, only he has regressed to a state where he can no longer function intellectually or take care of himself physically.

Alzheimer's disease is an even more precise diagnosis.

It is a particular form of senile dementia. In fact, many other things may cause an elderly person to become pathologically forgetful—to have senile dementia. There are Creutzfeldt-Jakob disease and multi-infarct dementia, for example. These are accompanied by brain changes that differ from those identified by Dr. Alzheimer. Alzheimer's disease is the form of senile dementia that is, among other things, invariably accompanied by profuse plaques and tangles, as seen in samples taken from the brain at autopsy.

As word of Dr. Alzheimer's work spread, more and more Alzheimer's disease was detected. Pathologists and scientists began to make an effort to look at brain samples from people like Uncle Joe after they died. Consistent with his demented jabbering at the TV, Uncle Joe's brain would be likely to exhibit many plaques and tangles, as well as considerable nerve cell loss. He had suffered Alzheimer's disease. So had a lot of others. In fact, through Dr. Alzheimer's efforts and those of the physicians and scientists who followed him, we have come to recognize that Alzheimer's disease is the most common form of senile dementia, accounting for some 70 to 80 percent of all cases.

More than this, we have come to recognize that Alzheimer's is not only the most common cause of senile dementia, it is common, period. It is estimated, for example, that nearly 7 million individuals in Western Europe, North America, and Japan alone presently suffer the disorder. Statistics vary from survey to survey, but an average over many studies suggests that 0.7 percent of those aged 60 to 64 years, 1.4 percent of those aged 65 to 69 years, 2.8 percent of those aged 70 to 74 years, 5.6 percent of those aged 75 to 79 years, 12.6 percent of those aged 80 to 85 years, 21.2 percent of those aged 85 to 89 years, and 38.6 percent of those aged 90 years and over are afflicted. Indeed, these numbers may be conservative. For instance, a widely cited survey recently performed in Boston found that 10 percent of the 65 year-olds examined had symptoms of Alzheimer's, a figure that rose steadily with age. A whopping 47 percent of the 85 year-olds had symptoms. Look your age group up in these tabular data and you'll see how lucky you are that you can even read this book!

These numbers also help explain why Alzheimer's now seems so common. No, Alzheimer's is not contagious; we aren't seeing the beginning of an epidemic—at least not in the classical sense. Rather, the statistics tell us that as we get older we become ever more likely to get Alzheimer's disease. Because the elderly are the most rapidly growing segment of our population, the frequency of Alzheimer's disease is increasing too. More elderly people, more Alzheimer's disease.

A second reason that Alzheimer's now seems so common is that it is not at all picky about its victims. Black folks, white folks, red folks, and yellow folks all get it. Rich or poor, you're susceptible. It is an ultimately democratic disorder. Indeed, as we now sadly know, Alzheimer's is not only democratic, it is Republican. There may be some minor exceptions to the relative risk for various segments of the population—for example, women are more susceptible to Alzheimer's than men even when you take into account the fact that women live longer than men—but these exceptions are so slight that they offer little reason to take heart or lose hope. The fact is, if you're human and plan on living a long time, Alzheimer's might well be your fate.

A final reason that Alzheimer's now seems so common is because physicians have become more knowledgeable about it and more comfortable making the diagnosis. Instead of writing down "senile dementia," or "senility," or some even less acceptable diagnosis such as "organic brain syndrome" (a $500 way of saying that there really is something wrong with your brain), they do a thorough evaluation and, when appropriate, they make the call: Alzheimer's.

This attention to better diagnosis has extended even to the death certificate in many cases. Previously, physicians of Alzheimer's patients tended to list only the technical cause of death. Most likely this would be either pneumonia or sepsis (systemic infection, here usually caused by bedsores). Alzheimer's patients are very susceptible to these problems because in the late stages of the disorder they become semi-comatose. As such, they do not clear their airways properly and the lungs become a perfect incubator for pneumonia and other respiratory illnesses. In addition, semi-comatose late-stage Alzheimer's patients don't turn themselves over in bed. Thus, they develop difficult to control bedsores, an infection that can spread throughout the entire body.

But the patients would not have had these problems had they not succumbed to Alzheimer's. As more and more physicians have become willing to make the diagnosis and to include Alzheimer's on the autopsy papers, our statistics gathering has become more accurate. We now have good reason to believe that Alzheimer's is something like the fourth leading cause of death among older adults. It's right up there with cancer, heart attacks, and car wrecks.

What Alzheimer's Disease Is Not

IN ADDITION TO KNOWING WHAT ALZHEIMER'S disease is, it may also be useful to point out a few things that it is not. It is not, for example, a movement disorder like Parkinson's disease or multiple sclerosis. Until the terminal stages, most Alzheimer's patients can get around just about as well as other people their age. They may forget how to do things or why they wanted to do them in the first place, but the muscles, bones, and nerve cells that subserve movement are remarkably unaffected.

Sometimes Alzheimer's occurs with other disorders and gives the appearance that it affects physical abilities. Parkinson's disease, for example, is another brain affliction that impairs the ability to initiate and continue voluntary movements. Muscles in the extremities may seem more rigid than usual and tremors may be observed as well. Because Parkinson's is, like Alzheimer's, an age-related disorder, the chances that the two may co-occur are increased.

Similarly, arthritis is more common in elderly people. If

it develops or worsens in an Alzheimer's patient, we might also get the mistaken impression that Alzheimer's is a cause of physical problems when in fact it is unlikely to be.

Compounding all this, as noted above, is the fact that Alzheimer's patients may be so impaired mentally that they have forgotten how to do even very simple things such as feed themselves. Or they may become so depressed and apathetic that they simply won't move.

The fact is that Alzheimer's strikes those areas of the brain that are associated with memory and other higher mental functions, while generally sparing the rest of the body, including brain areas that subserve physical activities such as breathing, heartbeat, and movement. Although my laboratory and others have occasionally noted a spread of Alzheimer's pathology to a few brain areas involved in movement, in my experience these changes are uncommon and tend to occur only in patients who have had the disease for a very long time. Thus, there are many other things that can co-occur with Alzheimer's disease and make Alzheimer's look like both a mental and physical disorder. But these are distinct and separate entities.

The general absence of movement and other physical problems in people with Alzheimer's disease has several medical and social implications. Medically, the development of such problems should alert the family that a checkup with the patient's physician is in order. The patient, for example, may be experiencing severe arthritis and in a lot of pain that he or she is unable to describe adequately to you.

Alternatively, the development of movement problems could signal that the patient has a disorder other than Alzheimer's. Creutzfeldt-Jakob disease, for example, has both physical and mental impairment as characteristics.

Socially, physical vigor in a cognitively disabled patient may actually create difficulties that require some creative caregiving on your part. You may have thought, for instance, that a lot of exercise was out of the question, but especially in the early stages of the disease it is not. In fact, it may be helpful in inducing that pleasant tiredness that leads naturally to sleep, something that often gets out of whack in Alzheimer's.

So, how long has it been since someone took addled old Uncle Joe, who used to be a regular member of the four-some, out golfing? Sure, at this point he may be unable to keep score very well. But did he ever in his youth? Just point him in the right direction. He may surprise you and knock it stiff. Similarly, an Alzheimer's patient who is accustomed to going out for a walk when he wants is not going to be pleased to be locked up. Uncle Joe would prob-ably get lost on his own and you may not always have the time, but there are alternatives.

What about Uncle Joe's old friends? Call them up. They probably want to help but don't know how. And you almost certainly will need the respite from caregiving as much as Uncle Joe needs the exercise.

In addition to not being a movement-related disease, Alzheimer's is also not "hardening of the arteries." This idea, common several decades ago, sprang from several sources. One of them was the finding that deposits similar to the senile plaques that characterize Alzheimer's disease are also often found surrounding blood vessels in the patient's brain. It was believed that the deposits, called amyloid angiopathy, impaired the vessels, and they probably do.

However, Alzheimer's disease can occur with little or no amyloid angiopathy. Atherosclerosis, a medical condition wherein blood flow is restricted because of clogging of the blood vessels, can also cause problems when the restricted blood flow is to the head. Again, however, many normal elderly people come to autopsy with tremendous occlusion of their brain vasculature and many Alzheimer's patients come to autopsy with little or none.

For these and other reasons, a vascular cause of Alzheimer's disease fell out of favor, although more recent studies, discussed in the next chapter, have returned to changes in blood vessels and blood flow as factors that may increase the risk of Alzheimer's even if they are not a cause. Whether they turn out to be significant in Alzheimer's or not, atherosclerosis, hypertension, and other vascular disorders are certainly to be avoided where possible. You have stopped smoking, haven't you?

Although there are some important similarities, Alzheimer's is not one of the prion diseases that have been so much in the headlines in the past few years. Prions are infectious particles, like viruses, but the mechanism of infection differs. Where a virus inserts its genetic material (DNA or RNA) into a host cell and induces the host cell to produce more virus, prions don't contain DNA or RNA. They are an abnormal form of a normal, non-toxic protein. Prions are infectious because when one of the abnormal forms encounters the normal form, the normal form is changed to the abnormal form. Each converted normal protein then becomes a nidus for converting other normal forms of protein. The abnormal protein increases exponentially, coalescing into aggregate deposits much like the amyloid deposits of Alzheimer's disease. In both cases, the deposits may be toxic. Alternatively, loss of the normal form of the prion protein occurs in parallel, and this could be equally or more deleterious to the cells.

Doctor Stanley Prusiner received the 1997 Nobel Prize in Medicine for discovering prions and how they are related to several nervous system disorders. The one you're most likely to have heard about is bovine spongiform encephalopathy, or "mad cow disease," which made its appearance in England a few years ago. The prion disorder most like Alzheimer's is Creutzfeldt-Jakob disease. Indeed, Creutzfeldt-Jakob has so many similarities—progressive dementia over a period of years, for example—that it is sometimes misdiagnosed as Alzheimer's. The main difference, of course, is that Creutzfeldt-Jakob disease is contagious. Fortunately, it's not easily communicated and is generally thought to require some mingling of the blood of an uninfected person with blood or other fluid from an infected patient.

An oral route of infection may also be possible, however, since mad cow disease seems most likely to be the result of contamination of cattle fodder with meat byproducts from other infected animals. In this case, the infected animals were probably sheep suffering from yet another prion disease called scrapie. Whether eating meat from an infected cow causes Creutzfeldt-Jakob disease remains controversial. The possibility has certainly not been good for the British cattle industry, however, and massive steps have been taken to insure that meat from prion-infected animals does not reach the market. Indeed, where prion-related disease has been found, whole herds have been destroyed so as to keep the infection from spreading. For what it's worth, mad cow disease has not been observed in the United States, so you can continue to enjoy your sirloin steak without fear.

Aside from clinical similarities, (for example, both are dementing disorders and tend to occur later in life) as well as similar staining properties of amyloid and prion deposits, Alzheimer's is not a prion disorder. Prions are not found in Alzheimer's brain samples, nor is there any well-accepted evidence of a viral cause of Alzheimer's. Alzheimer's disease is therefore not contagious.

Lastly, this chapter would not be complete without some mention of the notion that Alzheimer's disease is some form of behavioral disturbance brought on by mental sloth. In other words, Uncle Joe became a slug when he retired. He sat around watching TV all day long and his brain atrophied, so now he's got Alzheimer's disease.

Of all the things that Alzheimer's is not, this increasingly common misconception is the only one that gets my goat. One can readily understand confusion of Parkinson's or even atherosclerosis with Alzheimer's simply as the product of lack of knowledge about these disorders. But the idea that Alzheimer's patients are reaping the harvest of intellectual laziness requires an especially malicious human bent.

Where does it come from? As best I can determine after questioning recent audiences that have brought it up, it seems to follow from twisting certain scientific studies in ways that I'm sure their authors never intended. These studies are usually given as support for the "use it or lose it" theory, a concept that has been increasingly promulgated by geriatrician authors of popular books on "successful" aging. To age successfully, they say, you must stay mentally active because using your brain cells helps keep them and, more importantly, the connections they make with each other healthy. The ill-considered flipside to the argument, of course, is that if you're mentally lazy, your brain will suffer.

Now it's true that there are scientific experiments showing that prolonged stimulus deprivation can cause deleterious changes in the brain and in brain function. But these studies are mostly in rats and monkeys that have been completely isolated in small bare cages for a significant portion of their lives. To apply the results to adult human beings who have had a spouse and a TV and all the other implements and stimuli of a house for most of their lives is sheer nonsense.

Moreover, in my view and that of many other scientists, the theory should, if anything, be "use it and lose it," not "use it or lose it." For example, the more active a nerve cell is, the more energy it must burn. And the more energy it burns, the more toxic byproducts of energy metabolism it accumulates.

Alzheimer's is a disease. It devastates nerve cells of the brain just as surely as heart disease devastates muscle cells of the heart. With decreasing numbers of brain cells, you don't think so well anymore. Ronald Reagan did not get Alzheimer's disease by being a couch potato. On the contrary, this physically and intellectually vigorous man was forced into delegating his work and stumbling through his later press conferences by Alzheimer's disease, not the other way around. Similarly, Uncle Joe didn't get Alzheimer's disease because he sat around the house watching *Oprah*. With the increasing confusion of Alzheimer's disease, Ms. Winfrey's beautiful smile may have been one of the few things left that he could clearly understand.

Higher mental activity is the attribute that perhaps best characterizes us as human beings. It gives meaning to the phrase "quality of life." Of course you should keep as mentally active as you possibly can regardless of what theories are currently in vogue. Likewise, staying physically active and healthy is an important way to get more out of life whether you're young or you're old. But none of these things will protect you from Alzheimer's, nor will their absence cause it.

In summary, from these first two chapters you've learned quite a lot about what Alzheimer's disease is, and what it is not. It is the most common form of senile dementia—frighteningly so. It does not directly affect the patients physically; they can still get around and do lots of things, especially in the early stages. It does, however, cause impairment of memory and thinking so severe that the patient often can't make sense of the world, nor can he or she make sense to the world in many cases. It is associated with the same changes in the brain—plaques, tangles, and nerve cell loss—that Alzheimer himself first recognized some 90 years ago. It afflicts millions of people. All kinds of people.

And it's not their fault.

Who Is at Risk for Alzheimer's Disease

ALTHOUGH ALZHEIMER'S IS UBIQUITOUS, there are a few known factors that can put you at increased risk for the disorder. In approximate order of importance these are age, heredity, apolipoprotein E phenotype, prior history of head trauma, gender, and, possibly, vascular condition. Let's cover these in broad scope so as to prepare for the more detailed chapters that follow.

AGING

We've already summarized some of the statistics that show age to be the most important risk factor. For example, the average age of onset is around 65 to 75 years old, with increasing risk as the years mount. These are only averages, however, and there have been recorded cases of Alzheimer's as early as the late twenties. Conversely, my Great Aunt Mary Louise died in her late nineties as clear as a bell. Indeed, to her death she remained the only known person to win an argument with my father. Her technique was to conclude with the statement, "When you get to be as old as I am, you'll finally see that what I've said is true."

This, of course, was also my father's special last-ditch-argument-clincher; but with Great Aunt Mary Louise he was hopelessly outflanked.

The point is that there will always be exceptions to statistical averages. Some young people get Alzheimer's and some very old people don't. Nonetheless, on the average the older you get, the more at risk you become.

Why should this be so? Several reasons present themselves, although no one is quite certain yet how seriously to take them. One likely contributing factor is that nature has a great deal of difficulty protecting us from problems that occur after our reproductive years. Among generations of children susceptible to a particular disease, for instance, a mutation may arise conferring resistance. Individuals carrying the mutation will therefore be protected and will be more likely to survive. By being more likely to survive, these individuals will have a greater chance to produce children themselves—children who also will carry the mutation, have a greater chance to survive, and have an increased opportunity to pass along the protective mutation to yet another generation. In time, the mutation may spread throughout the populace in this way. The process is called natural selection, and we see it all the time in the histories of many different species.

When you think about it, however, natural selection has a tough time with diseases of the elderly. Individuals in our species may already have arisen with a beneficial mutation that protects them against Alzheimer's. As such, they will have a greater chance to survive their later years. But their later years aren't reproductive years; those days are behind them. Carrying a protective mutation against Alzheimer's will have no bearing on whether they survive to produce children or not, nor will it affect their children's chances to survive and produce offspring (even though their children also will have the beneficial gene). For this reason, a protective anti-Alzheimer's mutation is unlikely to spread through the population, and may even be lost. Aging may therefore be a risk factor in Alzheimer's disease because nature has been denied one of the primary mechanisms for protecting us once we get old: natural selection.

A second, more immediate basis for age as an Alzheimer's risk factor follows from the fact that Alzheimer's entails the loss of nerve cells and nerve cells are likely to be lost with age. This latter point is not without controversy, as it is very difficult to count nerve cells accurately, and even when we can we still don't know how many nerve cells were there when the patient was young. For this reason, several prominent neuroscientists have argued that there is little or no evidence for the loss of nerve cells with age.

I don't agree. To begin with, you only get the nerve cells you're born with. During infancy (or shortly thereafter for certain motor areas of the brain) the nerve cells stop multiplying. That means that every nerve cell in your brain is as old as you are. These cells are living entities, subject to random accident, fatigue and illness like all living things. If you're 70 years old, I doubt that you're as healthy as you were at 20, and I doubt your nerve cells are either. In fact, as noted earlier, the very energy processes that are necessary to keep nerve cells alive ultimately cause the buildup of toxic byproducts. Thus, to say that none of the billions of nerve cells in the brain are lost over the course of a lifetime is tantamount to saying that none of the billions of people in the world were lost over the same time period. Of course nerve cells die with age. The real issue is how many.

Equally important, and certainly less controversial, is the widely acknowledged fact that there is a significant age-related decline in the number of connections between nerve cells. These connections are called synapses, and losing them is probably far worse than losing nerve cells because nerve cells have to work in concert to get anything done at all.

Fortunately, of the billions of nerve cells and trillions of synapses we're each born with, not all are necessary to maintain normal function. I've seen children who had intractable epilepsy, for example, have nearly half their brains removed surgically in order to alleviate their seizures. Sounds barbaric, doesn't it? Yet, remarkably, many of these children appear to achieve normal mental function after they recover from surgery. Children are remarkably resilient.

Old people are not. Having lost nerve cells or synapses over many years, they stand ever closer to a precipice beyond which the accelerated further losses caused by

Alzheimer's disease are not so easily accommodated. In fact, Alzheimer's can lead to the destruction of as much as 50 percent of the large nerve cells in the higher mental centers of the cerebral cortex. In this view, then, aging isn't so much a cause of Alzheimer's as it is a susceptibility factor: when you're already near to that threshold where further nerve cell or synapse loss starts to have a tangible negative effect on cognitive function, it doesn't take much for Alzheimer's to tip the scales.

Just ask Uncle Joe.

Notice, however, that this hypothesis doesn't mean that just because you're old you'll get Alzheimer's disease. Aging kills nerve cells and nerve cell connections, and Alzheimer's kills nerve cells and nerve cell connections, but the two are not necessarily identical processes. With the normal amount of age-related loss, you may be able to survive for nearly a century or more without showing any obvious change (my Great Aunt Mary Louise, for instance). The destruction caused by Alzheimer's is much more dramatic. In an elderly person, add even the first stages of Alzheimer's, and you've got a problem that rapidly becomes obvious. Add Alzheimer's, in fact, and you can have a big problem even at an early age (the rare Alzheimer's patient in his or her thirties).

Recently, there has begun to emerge some limited, tangential evidence to support the above "threshold" theory of how normal aging and Alzheimer's disease interact. Several laboratories, including my own, have found, for example, that patients with very big brains can sometimes have enough Alzheimer's pathology (i.e., plaques and tangles) at autopsy to otherwise qualify for the diagnosis of Alzheimer's disease even though in life they showed no obvious symptoms. Since I wear a pea-sized 6¾ hat, I would never argue that a bigger brain will necessarily mean you're going to be smarter, but it is possible that people with bigger brains have more nerve cells and synapses. With more nerve cells and nerve cell connections to start with, such patients would be further away from that threshold where additional loss results in the expression of frank symptoms of Alzheimer's. Thus, in this interpretation, the patients may have the beginnings of Alzheimer's, but with a bigger margin of error (more nerve cells or synapses) they will take longer to show it.

A similar idea could also be garnered from studies that have attempted to relate intellectual ability to Alzheimer's risk. Recently, the Sisters of Notre Dame, an order of nuns in America, collectively made the wonderful gift of their brains at autopsy for Alzheimer's research. Their decision, I think, reflects the most powerful impulses not only of charity for the sick, but also of faith in an afterlife where the soul takes flight from its earthly body. In addition, they have made available certain personal records from each participant, including a narrative each sister periodically writes about her experiences as a novitiate, young, and senior nun. Examination of these records and the autopsied brains have suggested that sisters who had stronger cognitive skills (e.g., fluency and content of their writing) were less likely to die with brain symptoms of Alzheimer's disease. Assuming that the measures of cognitive skills reflect more nerve cells or connections between nerve cells (and this is a tall assumption), it could therefore be, once again, that starting farther away from the Alzheimer's threshold confers decreased risk or a delay in the onset of symptoms.

It also remains possible that there is a more direct association between aging and Alzheimer's disease than can presently be proven. The constant need for repair that occurs in the brain throughout life could eventually trigger processes that lead to Alzheimer's disease, for example.

At bottom, we do not know. Everything presented here, including my own views on age-related nerve cell and synapse loss, is at present mostly theory.

What we do know for sure is that your risk for Alzheimer's increases dramatically with each passing senior year.

HEAD INJURY

In addition to aging, another risk factor for Alzheimer's that may have its roots in the loss of nerve cells and synapses is prior head trauma. Although the surveys that have been conducted so far aren't terribly consistent with respect to the seriousness of the injury, or how long ago it occurred, there is nonetheless converging evidence that a blow to the head, particularly if it results in unconsciousness, predisposes one to Alzheimer's disease. Indeed, there is a form of senile dementia called dementia pugilistica that boxers are prone to.

If a head injury is severe enough, many nerve cells may be killed outright. In less severe cases, however, there is still substantial potential for damage. Head trauma, for example, causes a breakdown in something called the blood-brain barrier, a system wherein the blood vessels of the brain exclude almost everything from brain entry except oxygen and vital nutrients. Perhaps with head trauma something toxic is let into the brain that normally would not be.

Inflammation also frequently accompanies head trauma, and there is much evidence, covered later in the book, that inflammation is one of the causes of damage to the brain in Alzheimer's. Inflammation is an inherently destructive process that elsewhere in the body can be harnessed to play a beneficial role (though not always, as asthma and toxic shock syndrome readily show).

Certainly, inflammation of the brain is always a grave concern. Perhaps head trauma, then, sets the stage for an ever widening circle of inflammation that may later contribute to Alzheimer's.

APOLIPOPROTEIN E

As a risk factor, your apolipoprotein E phenotype may also play a role in Alzheimer's disease through the underlying basis of nerve cell or synapse loss. Apolipoprotein E is a normal molecule that everyone has. It appears to do lots of things for the body, including helping out with tissue repair.

As it happens, apolipoprotein E comes in three flavors: apolipoprotein E2, apolipoprotein E3, and apolipoprotein E4. The type of apolipoprotein E that you have is determined by the type that your parents had. It is hereditary.

Over the last decade, it has been shown that having apolipoprotein E4 instead of E2 or E3 can dramatically increase your risk of Alzheimer's disease. How it does so is not yet agreed on. For now, it may simply be worth noting that people who have both significant prior head trauma and who have inherited apolipoprotein E4 are at about 20 times more risk of developing Alzheimer's disease than other people their age. The fact that apolipoprotein E may play a role in tissue repair combined with the fact that head trauma usually requires tissue repair may take us back, then, to nerve cell or synapse loss as an underlying basis for these two risk factors.

OTHER HEREDITARY FACTORS

Apolipoprotein E is not the only thing that makes heredity one of the most important risk factors for Alzheimer's disease. To begin with, it is now clear that at least 5 to 10 percent of patients with Alzheimer's disease inherited it. The disease is exactly the same as in elderly people whose families showed no history of dementia, down to the same characteristic brain lesions. But when Alzheimer's runs in a family, there are some added dimensions. First, around 50 percent of the family will get it, generation after generation. Second, the age of onset is often earlier—on the average around 45, with some cases as early as the twenties. Last, and perhaps mercifully, the course of the disease is typically shorter, so that most patients die within about five years of the onset of symptoms.

The idea that hereditary Alzheimer's disease occurs earlier in life should set off some alarm bells in the common sense part of your brain. Consider, for example, my family. None of my blood relatives has ever been reported to have suffered Alzheimer's. Is this because the blood line is free of hereditary Alzheimer's disease?

Perhaps. Perhaps not. Looked at as a group, longevity is not a strong suit among my relatives. Many of us stroke out in our sixties. It may be, then, that we just don't live long enough for the Alzheimer's that is hereditary in the family to show up. Put another way, the earlier in life that Alzheimer's occurs in a family the easier it is to see that it's hereditary.

It may be that much more than 20 to 30 percent of Alzheimer's is inherited, but because the disease occurs later in some families we are less apt to see the hereditary pattern. Conversely, we may think that hereditary Alzheimer's disease is associated with an earlier age of onset simply because it's much easier to detect the hereditary pattern in families that have an earlier age of onset.

When this is taken into consideration, some scientists believe that as much as 50 percent of Alzheimer's disease may be hereditary, maybe even more. Whatever the exact percentage, it is certainly true that your genetic makeup is an important determinant of your chances to get Alzheimer's.

GENDER

A patient's sex is the final factor wherein some definitive risk for Alzheimer's has been established. There is a slightly greater chance of becoming an Alzheimer's victim if you are female than if you are male. Women, of course, live longer than men and so have more years—elderly years in this case—to develop Alzheimer's. Even when the statistics incorporate this greater female longevity, however, there is still a slightly greater risk of Alzheimer's dementia for females.

Why females are more apt to get Alzheimer's dementia than males is anyone's guess. My wife's favorite reason is that it's because females have to put up with males for so long that it just wears their brains out prematurely. A more scientific alternative is that estrogen may somehow help maintain the integrity of nerve cells. Because females lose estrogen late in life, they may lose more nerve cells.

You might object to this theory on the grounds that males never had estrogen to start with. That is, if not having estrogen causes nerve cell loss and Alzheimer's disease, why don't all males develop the disorder?

Actually, males do have small amounts of estrogen. It is provided to the brain by converting the male hormone testosterone into estrogen. According to the theory, this conversion process may continue in males even in late life, whereas elderly women do not have this route available for obtaining estrogen.

Anecdotal reports among gynecologists also occasionally suggest that estrogen therapy in postmenopausal women may be therapeutic for cognitive impairment, a result that may be indirectly supported by studies with laboratory animals. Alternatively, estrogen replacement therapy is serious business. Much work needs to be done before it could be recommended as an Alzheimer's treatment.

VASCULAR CHANGES

Although "hardening of the arteries" may not directly cause Alzheimer's, there is much to suggest that changes in blood vessels and blood flow can be contributing factors. Epidemiologic studies wherein many people are surveyed have begun to show, for example, that people with cardio-vascular disease, hypertension, or high cholesterol levels may develop Alzheimer's disease more frequently than people who do not suffer from these health problems. A type of brain scan called positron emission tomography (PET) also consistently reveals changes in blood flow in certain areas of the Alzheimer's brain. Moreover, as noted earlier in the book, brain blood vessels in Alzheimer's often are surrounded by deposits similar to those observed in senile plaques. When these vessels are examined more closely, they show abnormalities.

Vascular problems might contribute to Alzheimer's in several different ways. A connection with apolipoprotein E is one of the first things to consider because the main role of this molecule is to "chaperone" cholesterol. That is, apolipoprotein E binds to cholesterol, accompanies it through the circulatory system and helps direct it to where it's supposed to go. The E4 variant of apolipoprotein the "bad guy" in Alzheimer's disease, may also be something of a villain in cardiovascular disease because it's associated with higher total cholesterol levels.

Another consideration follows from the special treatment the brain typically receives compared to other organs. The brain is highly sensitive to oxygen deprivation, for example, and normally gets first call on oxygen in the blood. Subtle but chronic impairment of blood flow to and through the brain could therefore have a damaging cumulative impact. Moreover, the brain is shielded from many circulating toxins, including several that are released in cardiovascular disease, by a special lining of the brain blood vessels. Damage to the blood vessels of the brain could therefore allow entry of toxins, making the patient more vulnerable to Alzheimer's.

SUMMARY

To summarize, you are at increased risk of Alzheimer's disease if you are elderly, have blood relatives with the disorder, have a history of significant head trauma, are female, or are positive for apolipoprotein E4. Cardiovascular disease, hypertension, high cholesterol, and other vascular problems may also be involved. Combinations of these factors increase your risk.

No other definitive risk factors for Alzheimer's disease have received consensus acceptance, though many have been suggested. Indeed, in closing this chapter it may be worth going over some of the most popular misconceptions about Alzheimer's risk factors so that you'll have an idea not only of what you should be worried about but also what you can quit worrying about.

Of the latter, nutrition would be at the top of the list for me. I can't tell you how many well meaning people I have met who believe that eating bran, broccoli, and/or mega-doses of vitamins will prevent or cure Alzheimer's. And God help you if you eat meat!

In fact, scientists have been searching for such simple answers for decades, and they just do not appear to be there. Even aluminum, which has been so exhaustively studied as a risk factor that it warrants a later chapter all to itself, is probably not a cause of Alzheimer's disease. Eating a healthy diet, like keeping mentally and physically active, is always a good thing. Avoiding pollution and unnecessary pesticide exposure is beneficial.

None of these things, however, will save you from Alzheimer's disease.

What Happens to the Patient with Alzheimer's Disease

ALZHEIMER'S DISEASE BEGINS CLINICALLY WITH something that's familiar to all of us: forgetfulness. It's a joke at first, as it should be. Think of your memory as a filing cabinet. Every day you put new files in, and every year it gets progressively harder to find any particular file or to stuff a new file into the cabinet. It's normal that we become more forgetful as we grow older. We've got a lot more to remember! But with the Alzheimer's patient, soon something different begins to occur.

At some point, the patients begin to forget very ordinary but important things. Uncle Joe takes his usual afternoon walk in a neighborhood he's lived in for over fifty years, and he can't find his way home. That's one of the most common things that brings the potential Alzheimer's patient into the clinic for the first time.

Usually the family practitioner sees the patient first. He goes through a simple routine. Are you over 65? Do you know who you are, where you are, and when you are? If you do, you are considered to be "oriented times three," and you probably just had a bad day. If you are not oriented and you're old, you probably have Alzheimer's.

If the answer is the latter, you should seek a second opinion from a neurologist who has experience with geriatric cases. Don't worry that your family physician will feel threatened or insulted; he or she will likely second the motion. In fact, there are many reasons to seek an experienced neurologist's counsel, and few reasons not to.

On the negative side, there's the simple statistic that if you're over 65 and demented, there's a 70 percent or more probability that you have Alzheimer's. Multi-infarct dementia (MID) accounts for another 10 percent or so. It's a disease in which the patient suffers many very small strokes (blood clots in the brain) all the time. No one stroke is enough to cause the patient to lose consciousness or even know that it's occurring. But like a building with all the lights on, and someone going around turning off one light at a time, soon it gets pretty dark inside.

After MID and Alzheimer's, the rest of the causes of dementia in elderly people are pretty rare. So why should you go to the bother of having Uncle Joe checked out?

The main reason is that once every blue moon what appears to be Alzheimer's not only isn't, but is something treatable. Sometimes, for instance, elderly people can become so pathologically depressed that they withdraw from the world. They're so far down, they can't think straight anymore. If they're over 65, there's a good chance they'll be considered to be an Alzheimer's victim, despite the fact that with suitable antidepressant medication, they'll perk right up again. Similarly, there are a surprising number of our fathers and mothers who've gotten sufficiently bored with their retirement and the successes and failures of their offspring (dutifully reported every Sunday evening by long distance telephone calls) that they've quietly taken to the bottle. Hardly anyone may know about the patient's problem, but that bottle in the closet, given enough time, can lead to something called Wernicke-Korsakoff's syndrome. It also mimics many of the symptoms of Alzheimer's, and like severe senile depression, is treatable. With abstention from alcoholic beverages and vitamin B therapy many Wernicke-Korsakoff patients recover.

Alzheimer's patients don't. So make absolutely sure nothing has been missed, especially something treatable. Medicare should pay for almost 80 percent of a neurologist's opinion anyway, so why not ask for it?

At the neurologist's, Uncle Joe will receive a lot of tests. A CT or MRI scan should be done to look for, among other things, brain tumors that might cause the appearance of dementia. Brain scans and other tests may also help rule out MID. Certain motor problems will be probed to insure that the patient doesn't have Creutzfeldt-Jakob disease, a fatal, rare, and remotely transmissible disorder that otherwise has many characteristics of Alzheimer's. It's not terribly important for you to know exactly what all these tests are for. It is important that you know with as much certainty as possible that everything treatable has been ruled out.

Never settle for a diagnosis of "organic brain syndrome" or even "senile dementia." These are only expensive ways of saying that there's really something wrong and the physician doesn't want to stick his neck out about it. If pressed, a neurologist who has made this kind of diagnosis will quibble and argue that a clinical diagnosis of Alzheimer's cannot be made with certainty. That's true...sort of. There is presently no clinical test for determining with certainty whether a living patient has Alzheimer's. However, there are now several tests—tests for particular types of memory failure, changes seen with brain scans, fragments of Alzheimer's pathology in the cerebrospinal fluid, and apolipoprotein E type—that, taken together, can reach near certainty. Even in the most conservative view, the diagnosis of Alzheimer's can be made by exclusion. The neurologists rules out severe senile depression and alcoholism and everything else he or she can. When nothing else that reasonably can be tested is left, the diagnosis of probable Alzheimer's disease can, and in most cases should, be rendered.

The brain autopsy, after the patient has died, is the only certain way to render a diagnosis of Alzheimer's disease. Microscope slides will give the final verdict. But until then, a competent neurologist can make a clinical diagnosis and, if the appropriate tests are done, he or she should be right about 95 percent of the time by current statistics. So don't settle for less. Make sure that no test for a treatable illness has been left undone.

When the diagnosis of Alzheimer's has been made, you must prepare yourself for a long battle. In my opinion, this is one disease that's much harder for the family than for the patient. That's not to make light of nearly a decade during which perfectly ordinary, perhaps even extraordinarily bright human beings progress from their usual state to one similar to a newborn's. Rather it is to say that as the disease takes its cruel toll, the patients are progressively less able than ever to appreciate it.

At first the forgetfulness will be a worry even to the Alzheimer's victim. They may leave notes everywhere to remind themselves of the simplest responsibilities. Soon that will give way to a forgetfulness of the forgetfulness. It leads, in fact, to my own golden rule of diagnosis: if you think you've got Alzheimer's, you don't, and if you don't think you've got Alzheimer's, you do. At this stage, the patients will often deny that anything is wrong except the way they're being treated. The spouse, on the other hand, will insist that many things are wrong, quite possibly in the misguided belief that if only the patient would recognize that he or she had the disease then they would become more cooperative patients.

The care is hard, and grows progressively harder. On average, at about the fourth year or so, physical capabilities are still intact but mental capabilities may be so far gone that the patient cannot remember such things as "my pants go on the bottom of me and my shirt goes on top."

Uncle Joe may have the inhibitions of a three-year-old.

At this stage, in fact, he may not be particularly concerned if he has pants on at all. He also is 75, however, and still retains enough mental capacity to resent being treated like a child. He may not know his children, his neighbors, or his best friend. The woman who is handling the money in his wallet and who will not let him out for a walk on his own may appear to be a total stranger. The mildest man in town, deacon, Quaker, and scoutmaster, Uncle Joe may strike his wife of 50 years.

This or incontinence (loss of bladder or bowel control) leads to a new era of ruin. What had been merely emotional devastation for the family now often turns to financial devastation as well. Not to worry, you say. You have long-term health care coverage. Well, read the fine print. Until recently, few policies actually covered the major costs of Alzheimer's care. Most avoided paying by including a clause limiting benefits to "skilled care" (i.e., that provided by nurses and physicians). However, since there are only two approved Alzheimer's drugs for a nurse or physician to administer, skilled care isn't much of an issue for the day-to-day needs of Alzheimer's victims. It's custodial care they require, lots of it. The kind that a loving, 75 year old husband or wife will try heroically to perform, but in the end cannot. The kind that your long-term health care policy may still not provide, although many states, including my own, have added statutes to help protect against such abuses and many insurance companies have voluntarily adopted reforms.

The state typically won't help with funding until both

the victim and spouse are on welfare. Nursing homes are often good, but they are invariably expensive. There goes the retirement savings you spent a lifetime working for.

In the nursing home, no matter how expensive or sophisticated, it's my experience that Alzheimer's patients often take a fast downward course. There are lots of reasons for this. First, going downhill fast is what got the patient into the nursing home in the first place. The nursing homes catch the last stages of the disease, and so they take the rap. Second, in order to manage the patients, they are often put on tranquilizers. It may sound insensitive, but in many cases I agree with this policy (indeed, your family physician is most likely the one who orders the drugs, not the nursing home). The Alzheimer's patient at this stage often appears severely depressed and unhappy. Paranoid delusions are not uncommon. Although they may have the inhibitions and reason of a baby, these patients also usually have enough left upstairs to recognize that they're not at home anymore. It's a hospital setting no matter how hard the staff may try to make it appear not to be. I've seen many patients without tranquilizers just sit and cry all day, or bang their heads against the wall, or wander and jabber incoherently. In my opinion, there's no earthly justification for this suffering. Don't blame the nursing home for using tranquilizers. More often than not, it's the only humane thing to do.

Of course, tranquilizers don't do much for already badly failing mental faculties. Haldol or valium will make the best of us seem a little stupid. You can imagine, then, what they do to a late-stage Alzheimer's patient.

Around seven years from the first diagnosis or clear pathologic symptoms of the disease, most Alzheimer's patients will have become progressively mute. By the eighth year they take to their beds, curling up in the same fetal position in which they came into the world, and, mercifully, they die. The technical cause of death, as noted earlier, is usually either pneumonia or sepsis (generalized infection, here most often resulting from bedsores).

There can be considerable variability in the problems individual patients will have and the time frame over which the progression of their disease occurs. I have only given averages. Some Alzheimer's patients die within a few years of diagnosis, others more than a decade. Regardless, it is a sad history. In fact, I have yet to meet a family who in the end did not welcome the death of even the most beloved spouse. You must learn to forgive yourself that. The inexorably progressive dehumanization of the Alzheimer's victim is a darkness so deep that absolutely nothing good can be said of it, save that it is over.

What Happens to the Brain with Alzheimer's Disease

ALZHEIMER'S DISEASE DEVASTATES THE BRAIN, and it does so in particular ways and in particular brain areas. These are important things to know in detail if you want to be able to keep up with current research in Alzheimer's disease, or if you just want to know why your afflicted spouse, relative, or friend with Alzheimer's can't think straight anymore.

Let's begin with the major pathologic features of Alzheimer's. As you've already learned, the classic hallmarks of the disease are senile or neuritic plaques, neurofibrillary tangles, and loss of nerve cells.

Senile plaques were first identified by Alois Alzheimer. They are roughly spherical, microscopic lesions about 100μm in diameter (which is about one-tenth the thickness of the sheet of paper you're now reading). There are millions of senile plaques scattered throughout the brain of an Alzheimer's patient. The photographs at the end of the chapter show examples in a portion of the brain of a severely afflicted patient. Each of the black freckle-like objects is a plaque, and this is only a tiny area of the brain that has been magnified many times.

Senile plaques may contain many different things, some normal and some not. Among the latter are deposits of a molecule called amyloid ß peptide, abbreviated Aß. This molecule has come to have so much importance in Alzheimer's research that it's given an entire chapter to itself later in the book. For now, a few details will suffice. First, Aß begins as part of a larger molecule, the amyloid precursor protein (APP). APP is a normal molecule found in your brain, my brain, and the brain of an Alzheimer's patient. In our brains, however, the APP more or less sits around without doing harm. In fact we're not quite sure yet just what function APP normally has in normal people, but we do know that everyone has it.

In the Alzheimer's brain, for reasons that are now under intense study, Aß is released from APP and begins to clump together, molecule to molecule, eventually building up large fibrils. These clumps of Aß ultimately end up as insoluble (hard to break up) deposits much like grains of sand strewn all over the brain. They form the core of the senile plaque.

Surrounding the Aß core are other elements of the plaque. We find, for example, nerve fibers, many of which do not appear healthy. These nerve fibers are also called neurites, suggesting an alternative name, the neuritic plaque, that is more often used in contemporary research. Certain cell types in the brain, the glia, are additionally found within or just outside the margins of the neuritic plaque. The glia are not nerve cells. Rather, they are special cells that normally support nerve cells in many different ways. Within the plaque, however, the glia are typically altered in appearance. They may grow larger (hypertrophy) or they may begin to produce molecules related to attack.

Neuritic plaques are obviously not healthy areas of brain tissue, but they can be found at autopsy in normal elderly people known not to have exhibited symptoms of dementia in life. The difference is quantitative: Alzheimer's patients have millions of plaques; normal elderly patients have many fewer and sometimes none.

The second alteration that is characteristically observed in Alzheimer's brain samples is the neurofibrillary tangle (see photographs at the end of the chapter). Nerve cells each send out one or more fibers called axons to make contact with other nerve cells. In affected nerve cells, the nerve cell and its axons contain tiny thread-like filaments, neurofibrillary tangles. How these tangles arise is, like Aß, the subject of much research warranting a full chapter to itself. Similarly, tangles, like Aß deposits, can and do occur in normal elderly people, but not in the profusion seen in the Alzheimer's brain. Finally, like Aß deposits, tangles are clearly not the sign of healthy tissue. Indeed, in many instances the tangles can be seen as "tombstones," the only remains of nerve cells long since dead.

Over the past five years there has been considerable

quibbling among Alzheimer's scientists over the relative importance of senile plaques and neurofibrillary tangles. Some (usually those with grants to study the Aß in plaques) argue for the preeminence of plaques in the pathological hierarchy. Others (usually those with grants to study tangles) argue just the opposite. These debates often occupy substantial and precious time at scientific meetings, and in my view have been more of a monument to ego and self-interest than to a constructive resolution of issues. The fact is that plaques and tangles have been the defining hallmarks of Alzheimer's disease since Alois Alzheimer first noticed them in 1906. They are both associated with deteriorative changes in the Alzheimer's brain, and they are both extremely important to unravelling the mysteries of Alzheimer's disease.

In addition to plaques and tangles, loss of nerve cells has also come to be appreciated as a hallmark of Alzheimer's disease. This makes a lot of sense. With the loss of nerve cells you lose brain power. To preclude this, nature gives each of us an extra ration of nerve cells at birth, enough to get by to a ripe old age. Alzheimer's, however, takes away more nerve cells than nature could ever have planned for. As many as 50 percent of pyramidal cells, a pivotal nerve cell type, may be lost in certain critical areas of the brain.

With the loss of nerve cells goes a loss of the connections they made, and this is probably more important than the loss of the parent cells themselves. To think the simplest thought (or merely to wiggle your little finger for that matter) requires the concerted effort of millions of nerve cells. To achieve this coordination, connections with other nerve cells are made by nerve fibers called axons, which carry messages away from the cell, and dendrites, which receive messages and carry them to the cell. The point where axons and dendrites interact is called the synapse, and it's been estimated that on average each of the billions of nerve cells in your brain makes around 4,000 synaptic contacts with other cells. These connections appear to fare even less well than nerve cells in Alzheimer's disease. Thus, Dr. Robert Terry and Dr. Robert Katzman, two of the great figures in Alzheimer's research, have shown that rather than plaques, tangles, or the loss of nerve cells it is the loss of the connections between nerve cells that best correlates with the severity of dementia in Alzheimer's disease.

Very recently, a new hallmark of Alzheimer's disease may have been found by Dr. John Trojanowski, Dr. Virginia Lee, and their colleagues at the University of Pennsylvania. It is a lesion similar to the neuritic plaque and, like the neuritic plaque, appears to occur by the millions in the Alzheimer's brain. Because the new lesion does not contain Aß or react with the customary stains for plaques, it has gone unnoticed, despite its profuse expression, for nearly a century of Alzheimer's research. What causes it and what significance it has remain unknown. But stay tuned, because it's likely to be very important.

It is not just that plaques, tangles, nerve cell loss, and the loss of connections between nerve cells occur profusely in the Alzheimer's brain that is important for understanding why Alzheimer's is so devastating to higher mental function. It is also crucial to know where these changes occur. The brain is a large and complex organ. There are hundreds of named structures, and even one that's named for not having a name: the substantia innominata (the substance without a name). Some structures exhibit a lot of damage—plaques, tangles, nerve cell loss—in Alzheimer's disease. Others don't.

Lack of damage to the motor (muscle controlling) areas of the brain helps explain why most Alzheimer's patients usually maintain their physical abilities until the late stages of the disease. They can speak just as well; they're just confused about what to say. They can walk just as well; and indeed they will wander off great distances if left unattended. When we look at areas in the brain that are involved in movement and other motor functions, these typically aren't much impacted by Alzheimer's. By contrast, the structures that are involved in memory and higher mental function are often devastated. These higher centers include the neocortex (see illustrations), an area that is so highly developed in man that it covers over most of the rest of the brain. It also includes the limbic system, an area long known to be involved in memory.

A second reason scientists have been preoccupied with defining the extent of damage to the different brain structures in Alzheimer's disease is that it gives us clues to the disease process itself. There are established connections among the brain's different structures. Several investigators have shown that Alzheimer's pathology tends to follow certain of these connections, so that damage in one particular area accurately predicts damage in other areas connected with it (as well as lack of damage in structures not connected with it). From these hypotheses we have come to understand that Alzheimer's doesn't just arise randomly in the different parts of the brain. Perhaps damage in a few key structures induces damage in others with which they are connected. Perhaps there is even a spread of pathology along the nerve fibers that interconnect the brain.

Finally, we need to know what brain areas are most damaged by Alzheimer's disease because this tells us where we should look for the causative agent. Virus particles, for example, are hard to find even when you know where they are. Although a viral cause of Alzheimer's is widely discounted, knowing where to look for the microscopic changes that could underlie the disorder makes our research a lot simpler.

In summary, scientists have characterized Alzheimer's disease in terms of what it does to the brain and where. There are millions of neuritic plaques with Aß at their core. There are millions of neurofibrillary tangles. There is a tremendous loss of nerve cells and their connections. And these changes occur in precisely those areas of the brain that we know are important to higher mental function, the neocortical areas and limbic system.

No wonder Uncle Joe has such a tough time thinking.

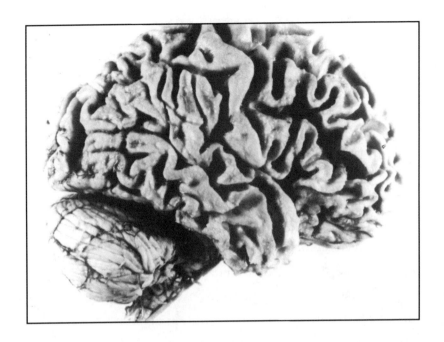

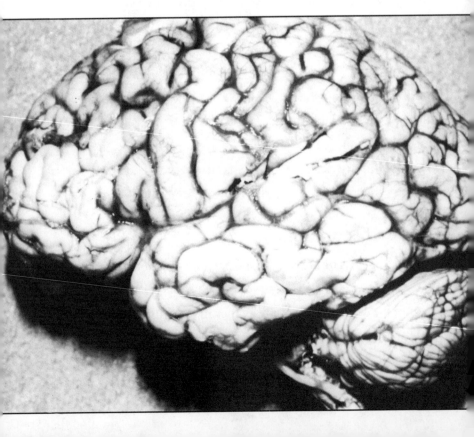

FIGURE 1

What Alzheimer's disease does to the brain. On the bottom is a typical brain that has been removed at autopsy from a normal elderly person. On the top is a typical brain from a severe Alzheimer's victim. Note how the Alzheimer's brain appears shrunken and atrophied. The convolutions of the brain, called gyri, are much thinner, and the spaces between them, called sulci, have widened. Presumably because some people start with very large brains, Alzheimer's changes aren't always as dramatic as here, but in my experience these examples are reasonably representative. (Photographs courtesy of Dr. Daron G. Davis, University of Kentucky, Dr. John C. Hunsaker, Division of Medical Examiner Services, Kentucky Justice Cabinet, and Dr. D. Larry Sparks, Sun Health Research Institute).

FRONTAL CORTEX

Ventricle

Basal Ganglia

Ventricle

Hippocampus

Entorhinial Cortex

TEMPORAL CORTEX

FIGURE 2

A typical Alzheimer's brain (left) and normal elderly brain (right) that have been cut to reveal some of the more vulnerable areas to Alzheimer's pathology. To understand where the cut was made, imagine slicing straight down from the top of the head at a point just in front of the ears. The frontal and temporal cortex, centers for higher mental processes such as memory and calculation, are highly affected, whereas motor areas such as the basal ganglia are relatively spared. The hippocampus and the entorhinal cortex of the temporal lobe are especially hard hit in Alzheimer's disease. Note that as the frontal cortex, hippocampus and entorhinal cortex atrophy, the ventricles (caverns where cerebrospinal fluid flows through the brain) become bigger, a very common finding. The optic tract runs along the bottom of the brain carrying signals to the primary visual cortex (which is at the far back of the brain and not seen at this level). Interestingly, the primary visual cortex often has some Alzheimer's damage, but not nearly so much as the higher visual areas in the temporal cortex. This is typical of Alzheimer's disease: as one progresses from brain areas involved in the receipt of lower level sensory information (the raw images of sight, for example) to brain areas involved in higher level processing of that information (what the images mean, for example), there is often an increasing amount of Alzheimer's pathology. Thus, although Alzheimer's patients may sometimes have increased physical difficulties with vision and hearing, their biggest problem is making sense of what they've seen and heard. (Photograph courtesy of Dr. W. Harold Civin and Dr. Alexander Roher, Sun Health Research Institute).

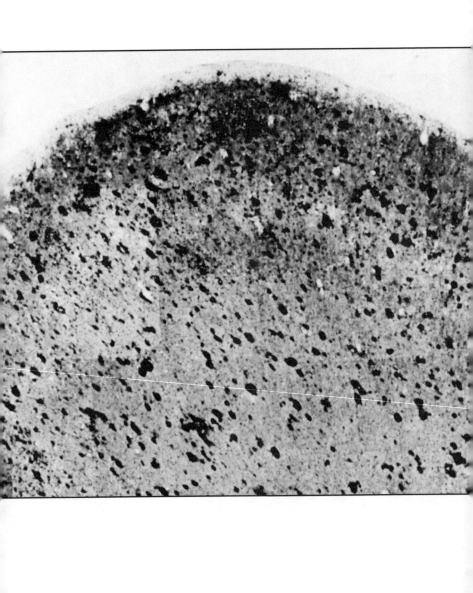

FIGURE 3

Photomicrograph (a photograph made through a microscope) at low magnification of senile plaques in the brain of an Alzheimer's victim. Each of the roughly spherical black dots is a plaque. Although this picture only encompasses an area of the frontal cortex about 1 centimeter square and 20 micrometers thick, there are several thousand plaques present. The frontal cortex is one of the brain areas involved in higher mental function. By contrast, brain areas involved in motor function have few or no plaques. (Photomicrograph courtesy of Dr. Alexander Roher, Sun Health Research Institute).

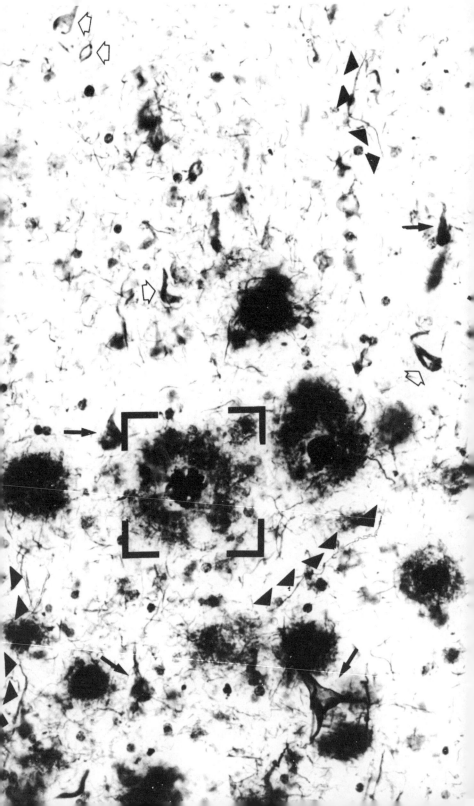

FIGURE 4

Higher magnification of frontal cortex brain tissue taken from an Alzheimer's victim at autopsy. This photomicrograph uses the same staining method to reveal Alzheimer's pathology that Dr. Alzheimer employed, and is probably very similar to what he first saw back in 1906. A typical senile or neuritic plaque is bracketed in the picture. We now know that the dense black material at the center of the plaque contains Aß. Surrounding this plaque core is a halo of deteriorating nerve fibers. Degenerating fibers not in plaques, called 'neuropil threads, can also be seen coursing throughout the sample (▲). In addition, numerous nerve cells containing neurofibrillary tangles are evident (→), some of which have deteriorated to the point where the only thing left of them is the tangle itself (⇒), the "tombstone tangle."

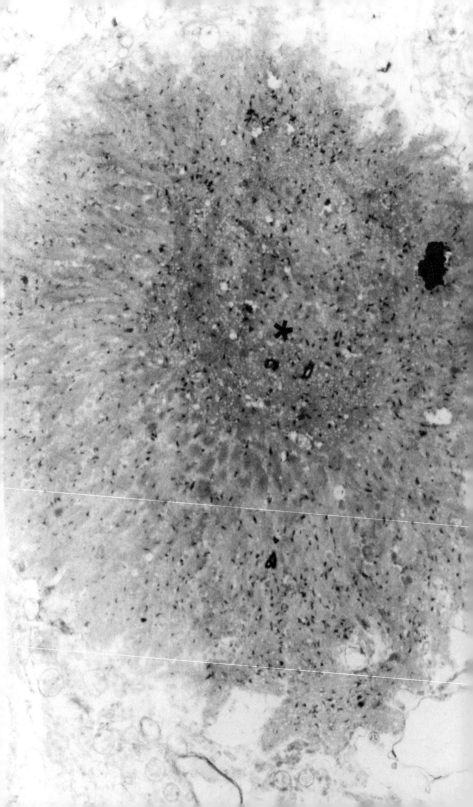

FIGURE 5

Higher magnification of an individual plaque. This stain, similar to that used by Dr. Alzheimer, reveals a compacted core of Aß surrounded by a rim of deteriorating nerve fibers. (Photomicrograph courtesy of Dr. Lih-Fen Lue, Sun Health Research Institute).

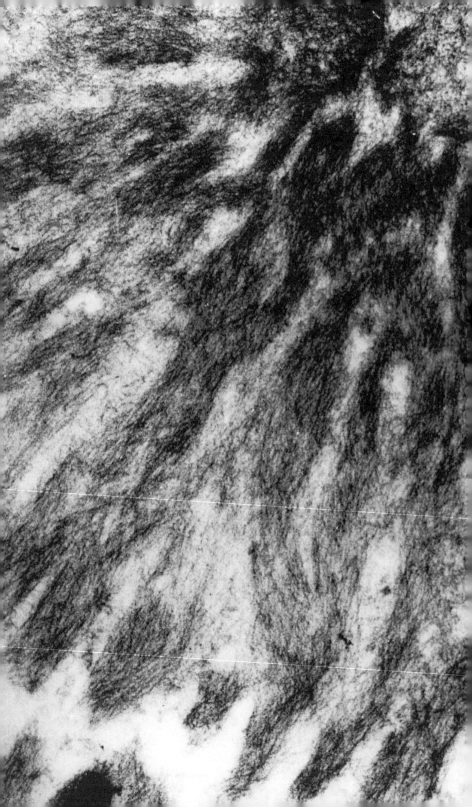

FIGURE 6

Photomicrograph of the center of a neuritic plaque taken with an electron microscope. Here, the plaque has been magnified many thousands of times to show how the Aß core (✳) is actually composed of millions of Aß fibrils. (Electron micrograph courtesy of Dr. Scott Webster, University of California at Irvine).

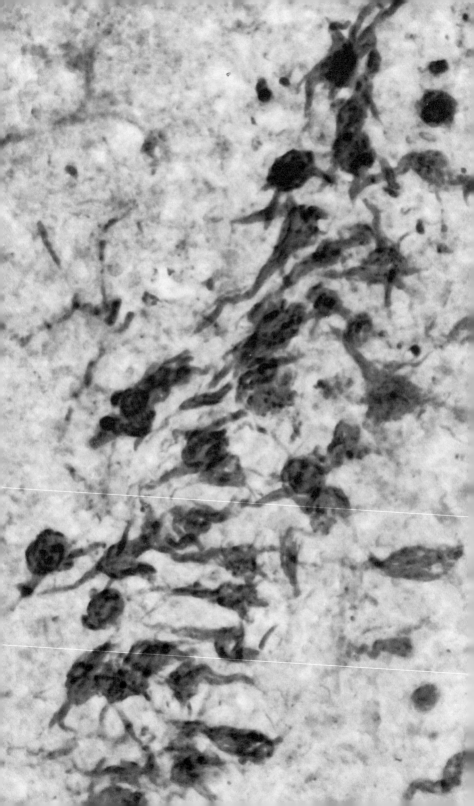

Figure 7

Like neuritic plaques, neurofibrillary tangles are profusely present in the Alzheimer's brain but are rare or absent in normal elderly people. Each nerve cell depicted here contains tangles—black, threadlike filaments that appear in the body of the cell and often extend into its processes. The region of the brain from which this sample was taken, the entorhinal cortex, is particularly pivotal for relaying messages involved in memory and higher mental function, and is especially vulnerable to neurofibrillary tangle formation. (Photomicrograph courtesy of Dr. Lih-Fen Lue, Sun Health Research Institute).

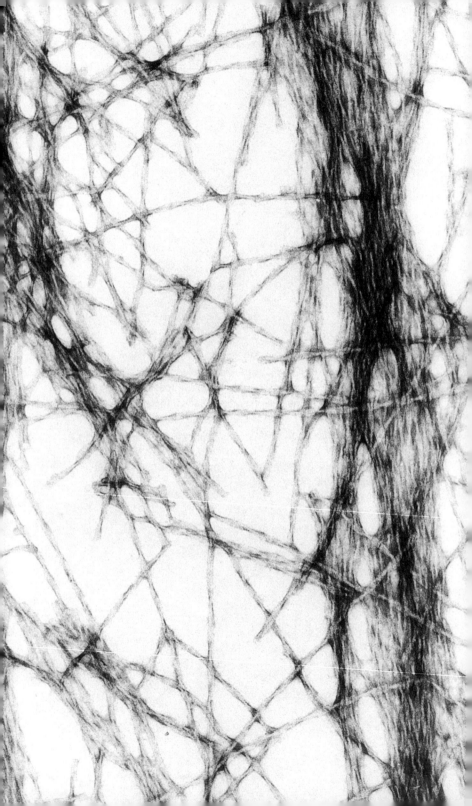

Figure 8

Photomicrograph of paired helical filaments that make up neurofibrillary tangles. As the name implies, the filaments occur in pairs with a periodic twist along their length. Paired helical filaments are so small that they can only be seen in an electron microscope. This image, for example, has been magnified several hundred thousand times. (Photomicrograph courtesy of Dr. Scott Webster, University of California at Irvine).

Acetylcholine

IN THE EARLY 1970'S IMPORTANT NEW GROUND was breached in the study of Alzheimer's. Dr. Peter Davies, at the Albert Einstein Medical School, discovered that a particular enzyme called choline acetyltransferase (abbreviated CAT or ChAT) was depleted by about 50 percent in the brains of Alzheimer's victims.

Choline acetyltransferase is an enzyme, a molecule that helps make the body's chemical reactions go. The reaction choline acetyltransferase makes go, indeed, is essential for, is the manufacture of a brain messenger molecule called acetylcholine (abbreviated ACh). When nerve cells that use this messenger want to communicate with another nerve cell, they first send an electric signal down their nerve fibers. At the ends of the fibers, there's a gap, the synapse. How does the message get across the gap to the next nerve cell in the chain? Acetylcholine. The electrical signal causes acetylcholine to be released. It floats across the synapse, fits itself into spaces of just the right shape, and causes the recipient nerve cell to start up another electrical signal (which travels to the end of its fibers, releases other messengers to float across other gaps to still more distant nerve cells, and so on).

Acetylcholine makes all this work, and choline acetyltransferase makes the acetylcholine. So, if you lose 50 percent of your choline acetyltransferase, you don't make as much acetylcholine, and messages don't get through.

At about the same time, Dr. J. Anthony Deutsch, Dr. David A. Drachman, and others were publishing data suggesting that drugs that interfere with acetylcholine disrupt memory. In addition, other investigators later found that a small area of the brain that contains most of the acetylcholine-containing cells is often severely damaged in Alzheimer's. The vulnerable structure is called the substantia innominata or nucleus basalis of Meynert. The names are unimportant (indeed, as previously noted, substantia innominata is Latin for the substance or place without a name), but the conclusions seemed inevitable. Alzheimer's disease disrupts the manufacture of acetylcholine. Disrupting acetylcholine disrupts memory. Therefore, the memory loss of Alzheimer's disease must be caused by the disruption of acetylcholine.

Unfortunately, the power of this line of reasoning seems to have been lost on the Alzheimer's patients themselves. Scores of clinical trials were organized using drugs that boosted acetylcholine. They are still going on to this day. A few successes were reported, but most of the trials appeared inconclusive or unsuccessful.

There are actually many reasons these days to believe that the acetylcholine theory of Alzheimer's disease, while important, is by no means a complete solution to the problem. Let's examine some of the reasons.

First, acetylcholine isn't the only chemical messenger nerve cells use to communicate with each other. There's a messenger called somatostatin, and another called norepinephrine, and around twenty more we know about, and probably another twenty we haven't even discovered yet. As we learn more and more about such molecules, including better and more accurate ways of measuring them, we find that they too are often depleted in Alzheimer's disease. So how can patching up just one chemical messenger straighten out the Alzheimer's victim? Most likely, we'd have to patch up somatostatin and norepinephrine and other such molecules as well.

Moreover, acetylcholine is only used by a percentage of all the nerve cells in the brain. Cells that don't use acetylcholine are also killed in Alzheimer's disease. What will providing new acetylcholine do for them? Not much. The converse is also true. Some scientists now consider claims about the severity of damage to the nucleus basalis of Meynert, the brain's acetylcholine center, to be somewhat exaggerated. An investigator at my institution, the Sun Health Research Institute, for example, found that the nucleus basalis, a major brain center for manufacturing acetylcholine, is sometimes just as badly damaged in Parkinson's disease patients who did not have symptoms of dementia as in Alzheimer's patients who were severely demented.

Lastly, many of the large cells in some of the brain's higher centers are lost in the course of Alzheimer's disease. These are among the cells that normally receive the acetylcholine message. What good, then, could it possibly do to boost acetylcholine if the cells that receive it are dead? The idea is about as sound as installing fifty new phones in your house so you won't miss any calls when you're not at home.

With two recent and notable exceptions, perhaps the most unfavorable evidence against the acetylcholine theory of Alzheimer's disease has come from clinical studies. Most of this work was initially undertaken with a drug called physostigmine, a compound that interferes with yet another enzyme called acetylcholinesterase (AChE). The job of acetylcholinesterase is to break down acetylcholine once it has carried its message to neighboring nerve cells. Without acetylcholinesterase, the message would just keep repeating over and over, tying the recipient nerve cells into something like a gridlock or terminal seizure. Under conditions where there's not enough acetylcholine, however, dampening acetylcholinesterase can be helpful: it ensures that what little acetylcholine is left will get across the synapse and deliver its message. If Alzheimer's disease were caused solely by the loss of acetylcholine, physostigmine should have worked. By and large, it didn't.

Other approaches were tried. Drugs that looked so much like acetylcholine that they could fool the recipient cells into responding as if real acetylcholine had been delivered were injected. These also didn't work.

A few years ago, a new drug that affects acetylcholine became available. Its scientific name is tetrahydroaminoacridine (THA) or tacrine, and its trade name is Cognex. Manufactured by Parke-Davis Pharmaceuticals, it has properties similar to those of physostigmine, except that it seems to really help some Alzheimer's victims. Why should this be so?

Part of the answer has been suggested to be that Cognex may be more active in the brain than physostigmine. You see, acetylcholine isn't just a messenger for cells inside the brain. It's also used by nerve cells that reach to the intestines, the heart, and other organs. When you give a drug that boosts acetylcholine in the brain, you also affect these other parts of the body. Your heart may race. You may have diarrhea, cramps, or worse. Given these side effects, perhaps we simply couldn't afford to administer enough physostigmine to do the job in the brain. Perhaps if Cognex is more active in the brain, a sufficient dose could be given. That was the hope because Cognex was initially reported to provoke fewer side effects than many of the other acetylcholine-affecting drugs.

Cognex was put into nationwide trials by Parke-Davis in the late 1980's. Unfortunately, concerns over a side effect of the drug soon emerged. In some patients damage to the liver appeared to occur at high Cognex doses, so the drug dose was reduced and frequent tests of liver function were inaugurated. Carefully weighing the risks against the potential benefit of finally being able to help Alzheimer's victims, the Parke-Davis scientists persisted, and were rewarded when the trial results began to come in. Although many patients did not seem to benefit, some unequivocally did. On that basis, the United States Food and Drug Administration (FDA) approved the use of Cognex as a treatment for Alzheimer's disease. It was the first time such approval had ever been granted.

In 1996, another acetylcholine-type drug called Aricept also received FDA approval for Alzheimer's. Manufactured by Pfizer, Aricept's mechanism of action is very similar to Cognex, but it has, in my view, some distinct advantages.[1]

First, you only have to give the drug once a day. Second, liver toxicity is not so great a concern with Aricept, so that you don't necessarily have to monitor liver function in the patient every two weeks.

The FDA is a very conservative body, as it should be. Their approval usually comes only after extensive testing in thousands of patients at a cost of millions of dollars. Does this mean that Cognex and Aricept are cures for Alzheimer's? No. Does it mean that Cognex and Aricept

---

1 In fact, I thought the advantages were so great that I went out and bought some Pfizer stock—which has done very well, thank you. This may be something you will want to take into consideration, however, given my recommendation of Pfizer's product, Aricept. Caveat emptor!

are completely safe? Not necessarily. Does it mean that they work? Maybe. Perhaps a little bit. For some people. Would I give it to my Uncle Joe? Yes. Despite the conservative tone that I've used throughout this chapter, unequivocally I would try Uncle Joe on Cognex or Aricept. Let me tell you why.

First and foremost, some limited success for Cognex and Aricept must be admitted even by skeptics such as I. That is, when I look at the data it is clear that some 15 to 20 percent of Cognex and Aricept patients show improvement. It's not a great deal of improvement—perhaps back to where the patient had been some six months ago—but this is much better than inexorable decline.

True, Cognex and Aricept are costly, and monitoring liver function, with Cognex, is literally and figuratively a pain. Even in the few patients who show improvement, it is only transient. Despite continuing to take Cognex, the patients once again usually go on their inexorable, progressive decline. Less information about long-term outcomes is available for Aricept. Perhaps it will be better in this regard. Right now, however, Cognex and Aricept are the only two drugs approved by the FDA as an Alzheimer's treatment, and this brings me to the second reason for trying them.

In my talks with Alzheimer's families I find that perhaps the most psychologically dispiriting thing about the disorder is the helplessness of it all. Now, with Cognex or Aricept, there is finally something you can do to fight back.

If you try Cognex or Aricept, and I recommend that you do, there is one important thing you should insist on that your physician may not think of. Make sure that immediately before the patient goes on the drug a thorough battery of memory and mental status tests are done. The minimum would be something called the Mini-Mental Status Exam, which your physician may be able to perform. Still better would be administration of the Alzheimer's Disease Assessment Scale by an experienced neuropsychologist. These tests are important because they are objective. Without them, families are usually so desperate to help the patient that they seize on the slightest small improvement (which can occur at random even without treatment) as evidence that the drug is working. You need an objective baseline with which to chart Uncle Joe's progress, and these tests should be repeated at least yearly. If the patient continues to go downhill much like an untreated patient, the tests will show it and you can then rationally decide whether you want to continue or not. Hopefully, however, your relative or friend will be one of the lucky ones. The chances may be less than 50/50, but those are still much better odds than doing nothing at all.

Aluminum

OUT IN THE PACIFIC ON THE ISLAND OF GUAM, there is a province where a native tribe, the Chammoros, live. It's reportedly a fairly primitive and remote locale, but it has attracted some of our best scientists in Alzheimer's research. The reason is that the natives there have a very high incidence of a disease that is unique to their tribe, and the disease has many characteristics in common with Alzheimer's.

The disease is called the Parkinsonian dementia of Guam, or Guamanian dementia. Like Alzheimer's, the probability of getting Guamanian dementia increases with age (though the age of onset is typically younger than in Alzheimer's), it causes a progressively worsening dementia, and the brains of its victims have neurofibrillary tangles similar to those found in Alzheimer's. Unlike Alzheimer's, movement disorders similar to those in Parkinson's disease also occur. And the incidence is very high—even higher than Alzheimer's.

Why this particular population of primitive natives

and, seemingly, no other in the world should get a disorder with characteristics of Alzheimer's seemed an intriguing and potentially informative question. Dr. Carlton Gajdusek, of the National Institutes of Health, was particularly interested. He had already won a Nobel Prize for figuring out the cause of another Alzheimer's-like disease, Kuru, in another obscure tribe (the cause, unpalatably enough, was eating brain tissue from a deceased relative with Kuru). Together with a team of scientists, Dr. Gajdusek set out for Guam.

They found that the Chammoro natives didn't perform ritual cannibalism, and so a Kuru-like cause didn't seem probable. After sifting through mounds of data, however, they did find one thing that appeared to be as unique about the Chammoros as the disease that ravaged them: the place where they lived appeared to have as much as five thousand times more aluminum in the soil and water than normal.

Dr. Daniel Perl, now with Mt. Sinai School of Medicine, asked to examine brain samples from the Guam patients. He found they had extraordinarily high concentrations of aluminum. Where was the aluminum being deposited? By outfitting his electron microscope with an X-ray diffraction apparatus to measure concentrations of metals, Dr. Perl was able both to visualize nerve cells in the brain and to measure how much aluminum they contained. He found that nerve cells exhibiting Alzheimer's-like pathology, neurofibrillary tangles, were where the excess aluminum was accumulating. In the same tissue samples, nerve cells that did not have any pathology (abnormalities) did not have excess aluminum. And this turned out to be true not only for Guamanian dementia, but also for Alzheimer's disease.

Since that remarkable discovery more than ten years ago, aluminum has continued to make headlines and has continued to be controversial. The main problem has always centered on the issue of cause or effect. You see, trace amounts of aluminum and other metals can normally be found in nerve cells. So the question is, did the excess aluminum get into the nerve cell and make it sick, or was the cell already so sick that it let in too much aluminum? One is cause, the other effect. If a cause, then perhaps we could cure Alzheimer's by getting rid of the aluminum. If merely an effect, there would be little point to doing so, for the damage would already have been done.

Lining up on the side of aluminum as a cause were a spate of research reports that quickly appeared. Dr. Donald MacLachlan showed that applying or injecting aluminum into rabbits' brains caused their nerve cells to develop pathology similar to neurofibrillary tangles. But the tangles weren't exactly the same as in Alzheimer's.

It was pointed out that patients undergoing kidney dialysis could develop an Alzheimer's-like dementia because their systems were being loaded with aluminum in the process. With time and the clearance of the excess aluminum, however, dialysis patients recover. Alzheimer's patients do not recover under any circumstances.

Aluminum refining workers in America were polled to find out if they had an abnormally high incidence of Alzheimer's disease. This is, after all, what one would expect if aluminum is a cause of the disease. It turns out they don't have more or less Alzheimer's than their friends who sell cars, work at banks, or perform scientific research. Then, to add to the confusion, a group in Scandinavia reported that workers there who had had extensive contact with aluminum on the job exhibited a slightly elevated incidence of Alzheimer's. Perhaps the bottom line is to stay in America if you're interested in aluminum refining.

Most recently, scientists in Great Britain compared the incidence of Alzheimer's disease in the various counties there with the amounts of aluminum in the water. They found a low, but consistently reliable correspondence: the more aluminum in the water, the more Alzheimer's.

To make things even more confusing, a re-examination of the water in Guam has suggested that the original investigators may have tested the wrong water supply, a source that the Chamorros have not used for many years. In addition, other hypotheses for the high incidence of neurodegenerative disease among the Chamorros have been put forward. For example, the Chamorros have been known to use the seeds of the cycad plant for food, and cycad seeds appear to contain a substance that is toxic to brain cells. In addition, it's been noted that virtually all the Chamorros spring from a very tight family tree that ultimately traces back to only five women. If only one of them had a genetic mutation predisposing to brain disorders, it might therefore spread rampantly throughout the population.

Quite frankly, the jury is still out on aluminum and Alzheimer's disease. Many scientists, myself included, believe that it might remotely contribute to the pathology of the disorder. But it is not the cause.

Let's hope this is the right answer, anyway. Because if it isn't, mankind is in big trouble. Aluminum is the fourth most abundant element on earth. It's in the soil, the water, and the foods that you eat. It's in the pots and pans you cook the food in. It's even in the antacid tablets you take when you've eaten too much. And if thinking about that makes you perspire, don't use a deodorant because they are typically loaded with aluminum.

Even with environmental efforts on a scale undreamed of today, we probably could not make a dent in aluminum exposure. So what can you do besides pray that aluminum doesn't cause Alzheimer's?

I have been asked this question so many times that I've developed some stock answers, though I try to be careful to note that they're more facetious than substantive. Following are some examples.

Take Tums for acid indigestion. It's one of the few antacids that doesn't use aluminum hydroxide as its active ingredient. Rather, Tums uses calcium carbonate (Rolaids has recently started doing this, too), and a little extra calcium might actually do your aging bones some good. But lest you think this is some form of gratis endorsement for Tums, or that they're paying me somehow, let me also hasten to add that I find them to be somewhat less effective for my stomach than aluminum hydroxide antacids. Your stomach now, your brain later—it probably won't make much difference anyway.

Likewise, my favorite cookware is aluminum. It spreads heat rapidly and evenly. Just don't cook acid foods with it. Acids leach aluminum out of the pot and into your tomato sauce. That this is bad for your brain isn't why I'm raising the issue. It's bad for your aluminum pots. They get pitted.

Lastly, you might search for an antiperspirant that doesn't contain aluminum. I don't know of one to endorse, but I'm told they exist. Just remember, after you've found your aluminum-free deodorant, cookware, and antacid, you've still only cut your aluminum exposure by a few thousandths of a percent. I doubt that will save you from Alzheimer's.

Heredity and Alzheimer's Disease

IT'S BEEN RECOGNIZED FOR MANY YEARS that in some cases Alzheimer's disease is hereditary or familial. That is, within a particular family Alzheimer's appears to be handed down from generation to generation.

At first it was believed that inherited or familial Alzheimer's was relatively rare—perhaps 5 percent of cases or less. In these instances, the hereditary nature was clear: around 50 percent of each generation became Alzheimer's victims, generation after generation. Otherwise, the brain lesions were the same, as were the clinical manifestations of the disease. The patients got progressively more demented, and finally died, just as in the presumably non-hereditary, sporadic form. The main difference, aside from the fact that so many people in the same family succumbed, was that the age of onset appeared to be younger. On the average, hereditary Alzheimer's was considered to strike at around age 45, whereas the average age for non-hereditary Alzheimer's was generally believed to be more like 65 to 75.

Today, for reasons that we briefly touched on earlier, it's believed that these estimates may have been too low. Too low with respect to the age of onset for inherited Alzheimer's disease and too low with respect to how often inherited Alzheimer's occurs. Broadening our previous example may help reinforce your understanding of how these underestimates might have arisen. Let's say, for example, that Family A has hereditary Alzheimer's. Uncle Joe started showing symptoms at age 48. A few years later, his younger brother also developed the disease, this time at age 47. Everyone already knew that Great Aunt Michelle had been senile, as had her sister, Uncle Joe's mother. When other family members in their forties, fifties, and sixties were surveyed, about half of them turned out to have dementia. To the scientists, physicians, and family, the verdict would be hereditary Alzheimer's.

Now consider another family. Here, the patriarch, Grandfather Warren, began showing symptoms of Alzheimer's at age 92. Is it hereditary? We can find out by examining his brothers and sisters and cousins. Of course, they will be almost as old or older than Grandfather Warren. The sisters, it turns out, died of heart disease in their seventies. One brother was hit by a bus at age 50. Cancer claimed a lot of the others in their sixties. Would they, like Grandfather Warren, have developed Alzheimer's if they had lived to be as old? We'll never know. From the available data, you certainly couldn't conclude that the family had hereditary Alzheimer's disease. But then, there's hardly any data to analyze. Everyone is already dead.

The point is, the hereditary nature of a disease becomes progressively easier to detect as the age of onset becomes progressively younger. If a family has an age of onset in the forties, it's easy to spot the genetic pattern because almost everyone lives long enough to show symptoms. That may be why we previously thought that hereditary Alzheimer's was characterized by an early age of onset: whenever we could clearly see a genetic pattern it was always in relatively young patients. But that doesn't mean that patients who get Alzheimer's in their eighties don't also have the inherited form. They may, but there won't be enough relatives who've lived long enough to show the pattern.

Similarly, we may also have to change our ideas about the frequency of hereditary Alzheimer's. Early ages of onset are relatively rare, amounting to only about 5 percent of cases. Previously, we had considered these cases alone to be the ones that exemplified the hereditary or genetic form of the disease. But if we admit that patients at much later ages may also have an hereditary form of Alzheimer's, then it becomes clear that the frequency of genetically determined Alzheimer's is probably much higher than 5 percent. Some scientists, in fact, believe that all Alzheimer's may be inherited.

Even for those of us who have spent entire careers

working on Alzheimer's disease, coming to grips with the new science of molecular genetics has been difficult. It will be for you too. Nonetheless, if there's anything in this book worth puzzling out it is the rest of this chapter on the molecular genetics of Alzheimer's disease. Striking advances have been made in this area, and you must understand it if you are to follow where much of the most important new Alzheimer's research is leading.

Let's begin, then, with a few basic facts about genes and what they mean to our lives. The body is built of cells and every cell in the body is built of molecules. The instructions for how to build each molecule are contained in the cell's genes. Each gene is like a blueprint for how to build a particular molecule, and the complete set of genes is like a complete set of blueprints for how to build a cell (indeed, any cell in the body).

Genes occur side-by-side in long strings called chromosomes. Humans have 23 pairs of chromosomes plus an additional chromosome pair (XX or XY) that determines sex. Within those chromosomes are all the instructions necessary to build all the molecules that make up all the cells of the human body. Some genes, for example, code for molecules that are part of the cells in your eyes. Some of these molecules, the visual pigment, may be blue, in which case you'll have blue eyes. Other genes provide a blueprint for molecules that determine what sex you will be. Still other genes are instructions for molecules that are necessary to build the walls of the cell itself, or to perform various housekeeping functions like absorbing nutrients to keep the cell going.

If you make a small change in a gene, you make a small change in the instructions for the molecule that gene is responsible for. Sometimes the result is trivial: you get brown molecules and brown eyes instead of blue molecules and blue eyes. Taken together, many such trivial changes add up to the sometimes large differences among human beings. Sometimes, however, the result of even a minor change in a gene leads to disaster: the molecule doesn't work properly. If the molecule is essential to life, you're in trouble. This is what happens, for instance, in a disease called phenylketonuria, which your baby should have been tested for at birth. Infants who suffer this disorder are born with a defective or missing gene that codes for a molecule that breaks down a nutrient (here, an amino acid) in food called phenylalanine. Without the gene, toxic products of phenylalanine build up and kill the baby.

Changes in genes, if they aren't lethal in infancy or childhood, are generally passed on to succeeding generations. That's why genes are considered to be the vessels of heredity. It's also why the very fact that Alzheimer's disease can be hereditary is such an important clue. It tells us that Alzheimer's involves genes. If not, Alzheimer's couldn't be handed down from generation to generation.

The connection between Alzheimer's disease and

genes has been followed up in a number of important ways. The first of these to pay substantial dividends was the discovery of a relationship between Down's syndrome and Alzheimer's. This research reads a lot like a detective story: certain facts were revealed, deductions were made about those facts, and a significant conclusion resulted. I'll give you the facts and let's see, based on what you've learned already about genes, if you're as good a detective as the scientists were.

Down's syndrome is caused by a genetic defect that leads to mental retardation (sometimes mild, sometimes severe) and changes in body appearance (sometimes mild, sometimes severe). The generally flattened face and a folding of the eyelids where they meet the tear ducts, normal in people of Asian descent, also occurs in Down's syndrome, leading to the scientifically incorrect and socially unacceptable term for the disorder, "mongolism." A better term is "Trisomy 21" because it states exactly what causes Down's syndrome. Instead of having a pair of chromosomes for chromosome 21, which is normal, Down's victims have three 21st chromosomes. With that extra copy of the 21st chromosome, the Down's patients also get an extra ration of the genes on the 21st chromosome. In essence, they have an extra set of genetic instructions for building certain molecules of the body.

Consider a very literal-minded builder who receives a set of blueprints in which, by accident, the plans for the 21st floor have been copied twice and included in the set.

He constructs an edifice with two 21st floors. This wouldn't necessarily be a tragedy except that ultimately it causes the specifications for the plumbing and many other materials to be off. By the time the top floor is reached, for example, the pipes are short of their mark. Everything has gone awry. Nature is also a very literal-minded builder. She tolerates extra genetic blueprints no better than a paucity of them. Down's syndrome is the result.

It has now been conclusively demonstrated that virtually all Down's syndrome patients over the age of 35 to 40 will show the brain changes of Alzheimer's disease at autopsy. They have Aß deposits, neuritic plaques, scattered throughout the higher brain centers, just like an Alzheimer's patient. They have neurofibrillary tangles in these areas, just like an Alzheimer's patient. They have nerve cell loss. Many are not simply retarded anymore, they are also demented, although it is controversial whether or not this behavioral change is as universal as the Alzheimer's-like brain changes themselves.

As alarming as these facts may be for those of us who have children with Down's syndrome, one can deduce a lot from them. You be the scientist. What genes should we be looking at and what might one of them provide the molecular instructions for?

Yes, you're right. We should be looking at the genes on chromosome 21, the genes that are duplicated in Down's syndrome, in order to learn more about

Alzheimer's disease. This is a very important shortcut. You see, one of the reasons molecular genetics may have been so long in coming to Alzheimer's research is the mammoth task of sorting through the millions of human genes to find out if one or two are defective. The task isn't analogous to finding a needle in a haystack. It's more like finding a needle in a haystack in the state of Iowa at harvest time.

Knowing where to look—the research on Down's syndrome—helped Dr. Peter Hyslop, Dr. John Hardy, and other investigators quite a bit in their search for a gene that might be involved in Alzheimer's. There, at the far end of the 21st chromosome, the chromosome that's at fault in Down's, they found a gene mutation in several families who had hereditary Alzheimer's disease. The gene coded for a molecule—a molecule that contains Aß, the stuff from which the senile or neuritic plaque is built. Thus, we now know exactly where the Aß that makes up neuritic plaques comes from, and we know that changes in the gene that codes for Aß can cause Alzheimer's disease.

What is perplexing is that this information still doesn't explain all hereditary Alzheimer's disease. In fact, only a small percentage of the families with hereditary Alzheimer's have a mutation on chromosome 21. There had to be, therefore, at least one other gene mutation to account for the remaining families.

In 1995, mutations in two other genes were, in fact, found. Mutations of a gene on chromosome 1 were discovered that accounted for hereditary Alzheimer's in a few more families. Mutations of a gene on chromosome 14 accounted for still more.

The protein molecule that is built according to the instructions contained in the chromosome 14 gene is called presenilin 1. Mutated changes in presenilin 1 lead to Alzheimer's disease earlier than any other gene abnormality, with an average age of onset of 45 years-old and individual cases as young as 35 years-old. The protein molecule coded for by the gene on chromosome 1 is called presenilin 2. Even though its gene is on a different chromosome—1 instead of 14—it looks a lot like presenilin 1, hence the shared name. Because of this homology (similarity), it's suspected that presenilin 1 and presenilin 2 play very similar roles in the body. Again, no one is quite sure what those roles may be, but there are some highly suggestive clues.

By looking at the structure of the molecules, for instance, it seems very likely that they are membrane proteins. Membranes are important parts of every cell. There's a membrane that covers the cell, a membrane inside that membrane that separates the genetic material from the rest of the cell, and still other membranes that separate certain specialized elements within the cell from each other. One of the latter is called the endoplasmic reticulum. Sophisticated techniques that allow us to see where a particular molecule is located in the cell consistently show the presenilins to be part of the endoplasmic reticulum. Because the molecule that contains

Aß, the pathologic material that forms senile plaques, is cycled through the endoplasmic reticulum, some scientists believe that the presenilin mutations somehow interact with Aß, perhaps to produce a more toxic form.

Another hypothesis currently under study is that the presenilins have something to do with a cellular process called apoptosis. Apoptosis is so complicated that scientists aren't even in agreement as to how to pronounce it. Some say a•póp•tosis, whereas others argue that it should be ápo•tosis. Whichever, it is a form of programmed cell death in which, on receipt of the right signals, a cell dutifully commits suicide. This is actually quite useful under certain circumstances, such as when too many cells of a particular type have been formed and the body needs to get rid of the excess. There is, for example, an apoptotic slaughter of nerve cells during normal gestation because, early on, too many nerve cells are always created. Apoptosis is also believed to occur in Alzheimer's, presumably as an abnormal process. Because recent studies have suggested that the presenilins might act normally to oppose apoptosis, it becomes possible that the mutated presenilins don't do their job very well: apoptosis is allowed to take place when it shouldn't.

Beyond the Aß and presenilin genes, the fact that Alzheimer's disease can be inherited at all gives us several other important clues about the disorder. First and foremost, it tells us that Alzheimer's can be caused, at least in part, by a genetic abnormality within our own bodies. This does not necessarily exclude other, non-genetic factors within or outside the body, because the Alzheimer's-causing abnormality that is inherited might still be one that is interactive with such other factors. Still, by understanding exactly what the hereditary abnormality that underlies familial Alzheimer's disease is, we should be able quickly to establish whether it is working alone or in interaction with other elements.

Perhaps more important, the identification of genes involved in hereditary Alzheimer's disease gives us clues as to how this disorder may arise and be treated in every-one, not simply those with the inherited form. Knowing, for example, that a change in the presenilin 1 gene can cause Alzheimer's suggests that cellular processes that involve the presenilin 1 molecule are likely to be critical to development of the disease even in people who don't carry the gene defect. We can then focus our research on these processes to learn more about what they do nor-mally and how they may go awry, whether from a defec-tive presenilin molecule in familial cases or some other mechanism in sporadic (non-genetic) cases.

Apolipoprotein E and the Susceptibility Genes

CHANGES IN THE GENES FOR Aß, PRESENILIN 1, and presenlin 2 are likely to account for almost all cases of Alzheimer's disease where the cause is an abnormal alteration or mutation in the genetic material. In these cases, approximately 50 percent of each generation will become Alzheimer's victims, the disease will strike earlier than usual, and the inheritance pattern is said to be "autosomal dominant." Recently, however, it has become increasingly apparent that genes can play a much more subtle role in hereditary Alzheimer's than is allowed by considering only the autosomal dominant cases where an abnormal or mutated gene is critically involved. Under the latter circumstance, because the genetic code is wrong, the molecules that are built according to the code will also be wrong. This is what has happened, for example, in families who have a mutation (abnormal change) in the genes that control Aß, presenilin 1 or presenilin 2.

But what if there should be several normal variants of

a gene. The genes that code for eye color, for instance, come in several different forms, all of which are considered normal. Likewise, we now know of three variants of a particular gene where one of the variants—though considered normal because it is widely spread throughout the human population—nonetheless confers increased vulnerability to Alzheimer's disease. This "susceptibility gene" turns out to account for many more cases of hereditary Alzheimer's than the autosomal dominant genes that were discussed in the previous chapter.

The first susceptibility gene for Alzheimer's was discovered at Duke University by Dr. Allen Roses, Dr. Warren Strittmatter, and their colleagues. It's located on chromosome 19 and the molecule it makes, apolipoprotein E, has already been identified. Everyone possesses apolipoprotein E. It and the gene that codes for it are quite normal. However, there turn out to be three normal variants (much like the normal genes that code for eye color can vary, producing different eye colors). The different apolipoprotein E types are apolipoprotein E2, apolipoprotein E3 and apolipoprotein E4.[2]

The apolipoprotein E type that you have is determined by the apolipoprotein E genes that you inherited from your mother and father. Your father might have given you, for instance, apolipoprotein E2 and you

---

2 I'm often asked what happened to apolipoprotein E1. Well, at first it was believed that there were four different apolipoproteins. Later, it was discovered that the first apolipoprotein wasn't an apolipoprotein at all, but by then scientists had become accustomed to referring to the second, third, and fourth apolipoproteins by their original numbers so they were retained.

mother apolipoprotein E3. Thus, there are actually six different apolipoprotein E types: apolipoprotein E2/E2, E2/E3/ E2/E4, E3/E3, E3/E4, and E4/E4 (the order doesn't make any difference, so that E2/E3 is the same, for example, as E3/E2).

Having even one E4 form of apolipoprotein E (E2/E4 or E3/E4) increases your risk of developing Alzheimer's disease or, put better, it appears to lower the age at which you might get it. Having a double dose of the E4 form (E4/E4) increases your risk even more.

Why should this be so?

We've already covered one hypothesis: the relationship of apolipoprotein E to cholesterol and cardiovascular disorders. The E4 variant is associated with higher cholesterol, which could pose many problems, both direct and indirect, for the brain. In turn, this could help set the stage for Alzheimer's disease.

Another current idea is that apolipoprotein E is somehow involved in the normal maintenance or repair of nerve cells, and that apolipoprotein E4 doesn't fulfill this function as well as the others, particularly E2. Given the extra ration of nerve cells we get at birth, this decreased ability to protect or repair nerve cells doesn't make much difference until you get old. Then, however, prior loss of nerve cells over the course of your life and a diminished ability to protect or repair them may have whittled down your nerve cell supply to a critical point. With apolipoprotein E4 this would occur sooner.

A third possibility is that apolipoprotein E4 interacts somehow with other elements of Alzheimer's disease to make things worse. For example, apolipoprotein E4 has been reported to stick to Aß better than E2 or E3. By doing so, apolipoprotein E4 may increase the chances or the rate that Aß molecules stick together to form neuritic plaques (recall that everyone has Aß floating around in their brains; it is only when the Aß clumps together that it forms neuritic plaques and becomes more dangerous). Consistent with this idea, Alzheimer's patients who are positive for apolipoprotein E4 tend to have more Aß deposits, senile or neuritic plaques, than patients who have the other apolipoprotein types. Through genetic engineering, certain strains of mice have been induced to form Aß deposits similar to those in Alzheimer's disease. Simultaneous removal or reduction of apolipoprotein E by further genetic engineering substantially reduces Aß deposits in the mice, further supporting interactions with Aß as a mechanism for apolipoprotein E influence on Alzheimer's susceptibility.

Still another hypothesis has to do with apolipoprotein interactions with tau, a major constituent of neurofibrillary tangles, the second classical hallmark of Alzheimer's disease. Here, the role of the apolipoproteins is turned on its head. All the apolipoproteins bind to tau, but apolipoprotein 2 and 3 do it better than apolipoprotein 4. This binding is believed to be advantageous because it helps keep tau from turning into a neurofibrillary tangle and killing the cell. Thus, in this view, it's not so much having apolipoprotein E4 that's the problem, it's that by having E4 you won't possess E2 or E3 and the resistance to tangle formation they confer.

There are likely to be susceptibility genes for Alzheimer's other than apolipoprotein E4. Dr. Roses and his group at Duke, for instance, have announced that there may be a susceptibility gene on chromosome 12, but they're still not sure of the exact location within chromosome 12. Among the 200 or so possible genes they've narrowed their search to, I find it interesting that right in the middle are two flanking genes that code for inflammatory molecules. It will be at least another year, however, before anyone is sure.

The hereditary basis of Alzheimer's disease, whether through an autosomal dominant mutation or a susceptibility gene, provides clues to how Alzheimer's might ultimately be treated. For example, if mutations in the Aß gene lead to Alzheimer's disease by causing massive deposits of Aß in the brain, then perhaps we might come up with some way to dissolve the deposits or prevent the Aß from clumping together in the first place. Further in the future, we might consider gene therapy, a scientific arena now in its infancy as far as human beings are concerned, but well established in plants and the lower animals. Here, it has been shown that a defective gene can sometimes be replaced or a new gene added to confer some desirable characteristic such as resistance to a par-

ticular pest. Perhaps using these methods we may some-
day be able to replace the mutated genes on chromosomes 1, 14, or 21 in afflicted Alzheimer's families who
have this problem.

In addition to helping us understand the causes of
Alzheimer's disease and suggesting cures for the future,
research into the hereditary or genetic basis of
Alzheimer's disease should also lead to a more immediate benefit. That is, from this work we should have a
clinical test that will help diagnose Alzheimer's in living
patients. This would be a great improvement because
presently, as noted earlier, the only way you can diagnose
Alzheimer's with certainty is after the patient dies. By
testing for genetic mutations on chromosomes 1, 14, and
21 we should be able to diagnose the major forms of
hereditary, autosomal dominant Alzheimer's disease. We
should also be able to test family members to determine
who is likely to become a victim in the future.

Demonstrating possession of a susceptibility gene
such as apolipoprotein E4 would also lend greater certainty that a patient's dementia was caused by
Alzheimer's disease and not some other disorder. Note,
however, that unlike the autosomal dominant mutations,
above, where possession of the abnormal gene confers a
near certainty of developing Alzheimer's, possession of a
susceptibility gene only confers greater risk. You may
have the susceptibility gene, but there's still a good
chance you'll never have Alzheimer's. For this reason,

the present consensus is that possession of a susceptibility gene should only play a role in diagnosis when a patient already shows symptoms. In this case, the susceptibility gene adds further certainty that the diagnosis of Alzheimer's rather than some other dementing disorder is correct.

If scientists can perform these genetic tests for their research, you might well ask why the tests aren't widely available to the public, especially families who potentially have hereditary Alzheimer's. One answer is the emotional anguish they might cause. Some physicians, in fact, don't even think normal elderly people should be told they possess a susceptibility gene because it will cause them to worry unnecessarily about a disease they might never get. Even with the autosomal dominant genes, where there is much higher certainty, one has only to read *Hannah's Heirs* by Dr. Daniel Pollen to become aware of the difficulties involved. This book begins with a beautiful and tragic account of a patient who knew he had an autosomal dominant mutation as he developed the early stages of Alzheimer's. Similarly, there has been for some time a genetic test that family members of Huntington's disease victims can take that will tell them if they're going to get the disorder. Perhaps not surprisingly, many decline.

A second factor hindering commercial development of Alzheimer's genetic tests is money. You'll recall that the autosomal dominant form is relatively rare—5 percent of cases or less. Manufacturing a test for just a few patients isn't cost effective, especially when there are doubts whether anyone will want to take it. The apolipoprotein E susceptibility gene and mutations in the presenilin 1 gene, however, can be tested. The test is available from Athena Neuroscience in South San Francisco, but it can only be ordered by a physician and only for the purpose of facilitating diagnosis of a patient who already shows symptoms of Alzheimer's disease.

In summary, should you be worried about hereditary Alzheimer's in your family? If one or two of your first-order blood relatives (mother, father, sister, brother) has Alzheimer's, there may be cause for concern, because it increases the chances that you (and your children) will develop the disorder by as much as two to four fold. Moreover, if your blood relative developed Alzheimer's while still relatively young, say in his or her forties or early fifties, your risk is even greater, because this may be the autosomal dominant form. Indeed, if you have had many blood relatives with Alzheimer's your risk can be quite high—as much as 50/50.

The problem for most families is the certainty of diagnosis for the other relatives. Alzheimer's, you may remember from earlier in the book, cannot be diagnosed with certainty except at autopsy. Moreover, several other diseases can cause dementia. Especially in your mother and father or grandmother and grandfather's time, all of these diseases tended to get lumped together as senility, and autopsies for Alzheimer's were rare. Thus, the probability is that the only data you'll have is that your living relative carries a clinical diagnosis of Alzheimer's, and one or more of that person's relatives died under circumstances that could have been Alzheimer's.

The answer to this problem, of course, is to make sure that an autopsy is conducted when Alzheimer's disease is suspected. There are a number of medical and research centers throughout the country where this can be done at little or no cost if you're lucky enough to live close by and are able to enroll the patient before death (so that clinical examinations can be performed). Failing this, an autopsy may be impractical, and the best thing you can do is to insure that a thorough clinical evaluation has been performed while the patient is living. As noted earlier, an experienced neurologist who uses the right tests will be correct in his diagnosis of Alzheimer's at least 90 percent or more of the time. That may be sufficient ultimately to establish whether or not there may be a genetic problem of concern to your family.

Amyloid ß Peptide

AMYLOID ß PEPTIDE, ABBREVIATED Aß, is probably the first thing Alois Alzheimer noticed when he began studying the disease named for him. It is the defining constituent of the neuritic plaque. Billions of Aß molecules clump together or aggregate to form the millions of neuritic plaques in the brains of Alzheimer's patients (see photographs on pages 62-66). For this reason, Aß has been intensely studied almost since Alzheimer's time. Despite its place in the history of Alzheimer's research, however, there is crucial information about Aß we are yet to learn.

Let's start with what we do know.

Aß is a molecule, a protein molecule. This means it is a complex substance built up from smaller molecules called amino acids. There are only a couple of dozen amino acids in nature, but these building blocks can be strung together like jewels on a necklace to create a nearly infinite number of different products. The instructions for how to string together the amino acids that make up a particular protein are coded for by the genes. One gene codes for one protein. Thus, as we have learned, there is a gene on human chromosome 21 that contains the instructions for how to string together the 40 or so amino acids that constitute Aß.

Of course, in reality it's more complicated than this. To begin with, the gene on chromosome 21 actually blueprints more than just Aß. It codes for a much larger molecule, about 700 amino acids in length, called the amyloid precursor protein, abbreviated APP. The machinery of the cell, under instructions from the APP gene, makes APP. This large molecule then appears to be transported to the cell surface where part of it is stuck in the cell membrane (the outer skin of the cell), with the rest of the molecule hanging outside. Perhaps not coincidentally, the place where APP protrudes through the cell surface is right where Aß is located.

APP may not sit hanging out of the cell for very long. Another protein molecule called α-secretase may come by and cut loose that part of APP that is outside the cell. Once released from the cell, the APP presumably floats around looking for something to do. What that something is, we're still not sure, but it's probably important. We suspect this because almost every animal species from lizards to humans has some form of APP. Moreover, almost every organ in your body, not just your brain, makes APP. Nature would not go to this trouble if APP didn't have some relatively important function.

Notice that when APP is released from the cell by α-secretase, the Aß molecule contained within APP is cut nearly in half. Under this circumstance there will be no intact Aß to clump together and form a neuritic plaque. Therefore, Alzheimer's disease cannot result because, by definition, there have to be millions of neuritic plaques in the patient's brain before Alzheimer's disease can be diagnosed. And millions of neuritic plaques require billions of Aß molecules to have aggregated together. No intact Aß, no Aß aggregates. No Aß aggregates, no neuritic plaques. No neuritic plaques, no diagnosis of Alzheimer's disease.

What happens if there is no α-secretase around at the time to release APP and cut Aß in half? It's now believed that an alternative route is invoked. Here, the APP is recycled back into the cell, broken down, and its constituent amino acids used over again to make other proteins (Nature, the mother of recycling, seldom wastes anything). Sometimes, however, the breakdown process may be incomplete, leaving intact Aß. The latter may be resistant to further degradation, especially if an Aß can quickly clump together with other Aß molecules. Such insoluble aggregates may be very unpalatable or even toxic to the cell. "Ptooey," they are spit out like a bad apple. Once outside the cell, other Aß molecules may join in forming a larger insoluble lump. The nidus of a plaque may be formed.

When we magnify a neuritic plaque thousands or

even hundreds of thousands of times using an electron microscope, the first thing that we see are the clumps of Aß. They form masses of fibrils (see photographs on pages 62-66). Coursing around and through the fibrils are nerve fibers, the processes by which nerve cells communicate with each other to think thoughts, hit baseballs, read books, and remember what has been read. Many of these nerve fibers appear damaged.

Perhaps the Aß fibrils are killing them. This seems possible based on research from a number of laboratories wherein nerve cells (usually from laboratory rats) are grown in test tubes under exposure to Aß. Many of the nerve cells are destroyed. Alternatively, Aß may simply attract other destructive processes. Certain specialized brain cells called glia, for example, appear to congregate within and around plaques. Some of these, the microglia, can become scavengers and attack. That they do so in plaques is shown by looking at them at even higher magnification. In their bellies, so to speak, we can see Aß fibrils and debris from dead nerve cells. The microglia quite literally have eaten this material. Perhaps the nerve cells were already dead, perhaps they were not—either is possible.

Multiple facts, then, tell us that Aß must be very important in Alzheimer's disease. Let's line these up.

The first point is simple history. Aß was probably the first thing Alois Alzheimer noticed when he "discovered" Alzheimer's disease. It has been intensely studied ever since. Indeed, the profuse presence of Aß is a defining characteristic of Alzheimer's. If you don't have it, you don't have Alzheimer's.

Second, the neuritic plaques made up of Aß can occupy a tremendous volume of the brain, as much as 50 percent by some estimates. Consider how well your brain would work if someone filled half of it with sawdust.

Third, it's not just that there's a lot of Aß around in the brain of an Alzheimer's patient, it's also where it is. The aggregates of Aß that make up neuritic plaques are found in precisely those brain regions where nerve cell destruction occurs, and these brain regions are precisely those that are known to be critical to higher mental function, the very process that is impaired in Alzheimer's disease.

Fourth, if we expose nerve cells to Aß they die.

Fifth, all Down's syndrome patients carry an extra gene for making Aß, and virtually all Down's syndrome patients over the age of 35 to 40 show massive deposits of Aß in their brains, just as Alzheimer's patients do.

Sixth, and perhaps most conclusive, if we alter the gene code for making Aß, we get hereditary Alzheimer's disease in the family.

Aß is clearly important to understand if we are to account for Alzheimer's disease. Surprisingly, however, not everyone agrees. Here are some of the reasons why. First, Aß deposits are almost invariably observed in autopsied brains from normal elderly people. You probably have a few Aß deposits and, based on my age (52) and wretched memory, I almost certainly do. Typically, however, the difference between the number of our Aß deposits and those of an Alzheimer's patient is so quantitatively great that it is almost a qualitative difference.

Second, a presumably normal elderly person occasionally comes to autopsy and is found to have profuse Aß deposits, just like Alzheimer's, yet there is no record of cognitive impairment. Perhaps these patients are so early in the course of the disease that not even our most sensitive memory tests could pick up the mental changes. Or perhaps these patients already had so much brain power that even the usual destruction of Alzheimer's disease still left them with enough nerve cells to function. A clue that this might be the case comes from Dr. Robert Terry and Dr. Robert Katzman, who were among the first to observe such patients. They found, as has my laboratory in independent studies, that such patients have significantly larger brains than other people their age. Aß could therefore still be doing its inexorable damage, but it would be many more years in these large-brained patients before enough nerve cells were destroyed to cross that threshold where normal mental function becomes progressively impaired.

A third argument against the importance of Aß follows from the fact that a certain kind of Aß deposit can be observed in areas of the Alzheimer's brain that do not exhibit nerve cell damage or clinical symptoms of

pathology. The cerebellum, for example, is a large structure at the back-bottom of your brain that is involved in
control of movement. Patients with Alzheimer's disease
do not show the kinds of problems with movement typical of patients with cerebellar damage, nor is there evidence of nerve cell loss in the cerebellum of Alzheimer's
patients. Nonetheless, Aß deposits occur there. They are
not, however, the usual kind seen in the higher brain
centers. In the cerebellum the Aß molecules clump
together in a different way from those in the higher centers, and their appearance is diffuse rather than compact.

Finally, there has been a continuing argument about
whether the extent of Aß deposition is correlated with
the extent of Alzheimer's dementia. One would expect
that the more Aß deposits present in the brain, the more
demented the patient would be. This was, in fact, suggested by a study reported nearly two decades ago, but
there have since been problems with the way the study
was conducted and interpreted.

Should one necessarily expect that there would be a
good correspondence between the severity of dementia
and the number of compact Aß deposits? In my view, the
answer is no. Recall, a few pages ago, our observation
that scavenger cells in the brains of Alzheimer's patients
appear attracted to Aß deposits and can be shown to contain Aß. The most parsimonious explanation is that the
scavenger cells are doing what they are supposed to do:
removing the Aß deposit. Thus, with time there is prob-

ably removal of Aß deposits through natural processes. Since nerve cells cannot be replaced, the damage done to nerve cells when the Aß was there will remain and will cumulate to produce more and more dementia even though, with progressive removal by scavenger cells, there may be less and less Aß to observe at autopsy.

A still better explanation is provided by a recent report from Dr. Carl Cotman and his colleagues, in which it is argued that what is critically important is where the Aß deposits occur. For example, in an area of the brain that is essential for interconnecting the higher centers that underlie memory and thinking, the entorhinal cortex, it turns out that there is a very good relationship between the amount of Aß deposited and the severity of dementia.

In summary, Aß is bad for the brain and Alzheimer's patients have lots of it in just the wrong places. So how can you avoid them?

The answer, so far at least, is that you can't. Without a fundamental understanding of why and how Aß forms toxic deposits in the Alzheimer's brain, it's difficult to come up with drugs to stop it. The only thing I can say that's hopeful is that we've learned more about this molecule in the past 10 years than in the previous 80 combined. It's my guess, in fact, that in the next 10 years we will have sufficient knowledge about Aß to rationally design drugs for it.

Neurofibrillary Tangles

WITHIN THE CELLS OF OUR BODIES IS A FINE meshwork of filaments that performs a variety of functions. It holds the cell together and helps gives it shape. It helps transport various materials such as nutrients to different parts of the cell.

Within many of the nerve cells in the Alzheimer's brain, an abnormal filamentous material arises called the neurofibrillary tangle. When stained with silver-containing chemicals neurofibrillary tangles turn black and can be readily observed with a microscope (see photographs on pages 62, 68 and 70). They are particularly prominent in regions of the brain associated with higher mental function and are generally not observed in brain regions that are spared the ravages of Alzheimer's disease.

Once formed, the neurofibrillary tangle is difficult to break down. This is true in the laboratory, where extremely harsh chemicals must be used to separate the different molecules that make up the tangle, and it appears to be true in nerve cells as well. In fact, we often see nerve cells in the Alzheimer's brain where nothing is left but the tangle. The rest of the cell has been eaten away leaving behind only a "tombstone tangle" where once the nerve cell existed (page 62).

The fact that we see so many tombstone tangles in brain samples from Alzheimer's victims tells us that the development of neurofibrillary tangles is likely to be toxic. Just how is not completely clear. Perhaps the neurofibrillary tangles are an abnormal variant of normal filaments but don't work as well. In that case, the cell might starve because essential nutrients and other materials can't be properly transported to the places where they're needed. Perhaps they interfere with the function of normal neurofilaments. You'd get the same unhappy result.

What the neurofibrillary tangle is composed of is also not completely clear. When viewed under the electron microscope, which magnifies thousands of times more than the light microscope Dr. Alzheimer had available to him, neurofibrillary tangles appear to contain tiny twisted rods called paired helical filaments (page 70). A molecule called tau is widely believed to be one of the constituents of paired helical filaments, but the rest is subject to seemingly endless debate. In part this is because whenever you try to isolate tangles or paired helical filaments it's difficult to be sure that you haven't lost part of them in the process or, just as bad, managed to contaminate the sample with other materials that were present in the brain tissue you're working with. Some neurofibrillary tangle preparations, for example, contain Aß. Was this there before or did some nearby Aß deposits get mixed up with the tangles in the isolation procedure?

Another constituent of tangles that has recently emerged is a glycolipid whose structure has not been completely resolved. Glycolipids are macromolecules (complexes of different molecules) containing different kinds of sugar and fatty acids.

Finally, how neurofibrillary tangles form in the first place remains unknown, but new clues have begun to emerge. Most of the research focuses on tau. Tau is present in normal neurofilaments and, as noted above, is one of the few molecules that most scientists agree is a constituent of tangles. Like many normal molecules, tau has a number of phosphate molecules attached to it. In Alzheimer's disease new evidence suggests that the tau in nerve cells may become hyperphosphorylated. That is, it has too many phosphate molecules, the presence of which may disrupt the normal function of tau and cause the normal neurofilaments that contain it to become abnormal paired helical filaments. This, in turn, causes the formation of neurofibrillary tangles.

Perhaps the best evidence for a role of hyperphosphorylated tau in tangle formation is the fact that when put in a test tube all by itself it forms filaments that are very similar to the paired helical or tangle filaments in the Alzheimer's brain. However, the tangle glycolipid that has recently been discovered also forms filaments in a test tube. Moreover, whereas the tau in normal adults isn't hyperphosphorylated, it is in the fetal brain. Since we don't see neurofibrillary tangles in fetal brain samples, the role of hyperphosphorylated tau in tangle formation becomes problematic.

Some investigators believe that Aß may cause neurofibrillary tangles to form, or vice-versa, although studies in my laboratory and others have not been particularly supportive. We counted, for example, Aß deposits and tangles in several different brain regions over many different patients, seeking a correlation between the two. That is, if Aß deposits cause tangles (or tangles cause Aß deposits), then you'd expect that as the number of one went up, the number of the other would go up in parallel. We didn't find anything of the kind.

It has also been suggested that reactive oxygen species play a role in tangle formation. Cells use oxygen in order to gain the energy necessary to keep them going, and this ultimately causes a buildup of toxic oxygen byproducts, the reactive oxygen species. Hydrogen peroxide is an example of a reactive oxygen species with which you're already familiar. You pour it on a wound to kill bacterial cells that may have entered the cut. Likewise, hydrogen peroxide and other reactive oxygen species that are produced in the brain can kill brain cells.

In Alzheimer's disease there is evidence that reactive oxygen species can combine with tau and cause it to form tangle-like filaments, as well as add extra phosphate molecules to form hyperphosphorylated tau. Moreover, when tau and reactive oxygen species are put together they may form an even more toxic molecule than either alone.

The number of neurofibrillary tangles found in an Alzheimer's patient's brain correlates somewhat with how demented the patient is. For reasons mentioned in the last chapter, tangles are, in fact, a better predictor of the severity of Alzheimer's disease than Aß deposits, though neither is as good a measure as the loss of nerve cells or the connections between nerve cells. The amount of tau present in the cerebrospinal fluid is also used in diagnostic tests for Alzheimer's disease. Though not infallible, a positive test can lend further weight to the diagnosis of Alzheimer's as opposed to some other dementing disorder.

What can be done about neurofibrillary tangles? How can you keep them from forming in your brain? Presently, the only viable option is to take anti-oxidants like vitamin E—assuming, of course, that the reactive oxygen species theory is correct, which it may not be. The good news is that vitamin E is unlikely to hurt you unless you do something silly like take a half dozen pills a day. Your body probably won't absorb any more than the standard 200-400 IU dose anyway, so stick with that and hope it works.

Inflammation

WHAT MAKES Aß AND NEUROFIBRILLARY tangles so bad for the brain? In fact, there are several potential mechanisms, no one of which may be primary. Among them is inflammation. Because the role of inflammation and Alzheimer's disease is a research area that my laboratory helped pioneer, I may be a bit biased about the importance of this topic. I'll try to lay the facts out objectively and let you be the judge.

In addition to Aß deposits, damaged and undamaged nerve fibers, and glia, neuritic plaques contain other elements. In particular, when we look carefully at the area within plaques that surrounds Aß deposits we find almost all the same inflammatory molecules that are present in an arthritic joint or the inflamed tissue where you've cut your finger. Likewise, there is now evidence that inflammation may occur in the context of neurofibrillary tangles, the second pathologic hallmark of Alzheimer's.

Inflammation is an inherently destructive set of

mechanisms that your body uses to advantage in the healing process. Your cut finger may contain dirt and bacteria, skin and other cells damaged by the wound, and infected tissue. To get rid of them, molecular messages were sent out when your finger was nicked ordering the production of inflammatory molecules locally or signalling their recruitment from the bloodstream. These inflammatory molecules have diverse tasks. Some activate scavenger cells to get busy. Others mark the dirt, bacteria, and cells killed or damaged in the accident so that the scavenger cells will have an easier time finding them. Still other inflammatory molecules directly attack the wound itself.

If all goes well, the area that's been hurt will be cleansed of almost everything in sight, including a few healthy cells that were in the way. This is no problem, however, because you can just grow some new skin cells to replace the old. Our bodies do this constantly in any case. In addition, at almost the same time the need for inflammation was signalled, a second, slower set of molecular messages was generated. These latter messages put the brakes on inflammation and ultimately halt it. A scab forms over the formerly red, inflamed cut, with new cells growing underneath to replace the old. Inflammation is halted. Thanks to inflammation, you're good as new.

That is, assuming that the inflammatory mechanisms worked properly. Inflammation can go awry.

Asthma, for example, occurs when the airways become inflamed due to what should have been only an innocuous challenge such as the inhalation of a pollen or the dander from a cat. Arthritis is another example. Here, inflammation continually attacks what should be normal tissue in the joints. Given enough time, the joint may be completely destroyed.

Alzheimer's disease may have in common with these disorders a perverse inflammatory attack. And more than this, the inflammatory attack could not be in a worse place. The simple inflammatory swelling that you experienced in your cut finger can be deadly in the brain because the nervous system is so neatly encapsulated by the skull there's no room for it to swell. Worse still, unlike skin and other cells, nerve cells cannot be replaced. All the nerve cells you will ever receive have been with you since childhood. If inflammatory reactions kill some of them, they are gone forever. For these and other reasons, inflammation is always a grave concern whenever it arises in the brain.

The Alzheimer's brain may be especially vulnerable in this regard. If every plaque and tangle is a potential nidus for inflammation, then the profusion of these pathologic hallmarks in the Alzheimer's brain means that the extent of inflammation there is probably substantial, even if each inflammatory site is itself microscopic. Notice, too, that things are likely to get worse. The damage to nerve cells and nerve fibers that Aß and neurofibrillary tangles are known to cause will breed inflammation. Inflammation may then damage more nerve cells and fibers. This will invoke still more inflammation. A vicious cycle may ensue. At first the problem may be minor: we have millions of nerve cells and billions of nerve fibers to spare. Cumulated over a decade, however, the problem may become substantial. Just ask anyone who's had arthritic inflammation eating away their knee or hip joints for the past few years.

Beyond these traditional scenarios for inflammatory destruction, inflammation may also interact with Alzheimer's pathology in a number of uniquely detrimental ways that it does not in other parts of the body or in other disease states. For example, complement, a set of inflammatory molecules that can kill cells, is usually only brought into play by very specific circumstances such as invasion of the body by a bacterium. However, complement is also activated by Aß. The nerve fibers that course through Aß deposits can thereby become a target for complement attack.

In addition, a particular complement molecule called C1q may play a role in the aggregation of Aß into its toxic state. As noted earlier, all of us have Aß in our brains. In the Alzheimer's brain, however, the Aß clumps together into the insoluble deposits that form neuritic plaques. C1q may help explain why this occurs. Our studies show that when C1q is present, Aß clumps together at some seven to ten times the rate that it normally does. Other molecules have been reported to do this as well—apolipoprotein E, for example. In our experience, however, none of these are as effective in binding Aß together into its toxic form as the inflammatory molecule C1q.

In addition to complement and the activation of scavenger cells, inflammation has other mechanisms available for doing damage to the brain. Another set of molecules called cytokines is released in the inflammatory process. These, too, can have much destructive potential. One of them, in fact, has been shown in vitro (in a test tube) to stimulate the APP gene, potentially liberating more Aß to form more plaques to serve as the nidus for more inflammation—yet another vicious cycle that inflammation in the Alzheimer's brain may spawn.

Despite these observations, some scientists still do not believe that inflammation plays an important role in Alzheimer's disease. Although they do not question that it occurs, they argue that inflammation is only present in order to remove the detritus left behind by the real causes of Alzheimer's (whatever these might be). Inflammation in and of itself does not kill nerve cells.

I do not agree with this point of view for several reasons, and the first reason is one that you can now probably recognize better than my scientist adversaries: inflammation is inherently destructive. Yes, that destructiveness can be harnessed to advantage in other parts of the body, but seldom in the brain. It is nearly axiomatic that any inflammation occurring in the brain will kill nerve cells. This can, in fact, be seen directly in the brains of Alzheimer's patients. Take a look at the photograph on the last page of this chapter. What you're seeing is a nerve fiber in the vicinity of an Aß deposit. Notice the big holes in the membrane (outer covering) of the fiber and the little black dots (arrows) there. These little black dots are a chemical marker for an inflammatory molecule called the membrane attack complex. As you can see, the molecule is aptly named. It binds to the cell membrane and blows open a hole there. The cell tries to defend itself by shedding the damaged area (➜) or internalizing it (⇨) where it can be harmlessly broken down. If enough membrane attack molecules are present, as is almost certainly the case here, the defense is to no avail. This nerve fiber is doomed to die by inflammation.

We can also show, using other methods, that the interactions of Aß with inflammation directly kill nerve cells. For example, when rat nerve cells are grown in a test tube and exposed to Aß, many of the cells die. However, if inflammation is allowed to take place as well, many more nerve cells die and it takes thousands of times less Aß to do it.

We have noted that Aß deposits occur in the cerebellum of Alzheimer's patients, but that this brain structure, unlike the higher brain centers, does not appear damaged. Why not? One reason may be that inflammation does not appear to occur in the Alzheimer's cerebellum.

Thus, when we look at Aß deposits in the higher centers we find profuse evidence of inflammation. When we look at Aß deposits in the cerebellum, we find little if any evidence of inflammation.

We also noted that occasionally normal elderly patients show up at autopsy with millions of Aß deposits and thousands of neurofibrillary tangles, but in life they evidenced little apparent problem with their memory or thinking. Why not? When we look at Aß deposits and neurofibrillary tangles in the higher brain centers of Alzheimer's patients, we see profuse evidence of inflammation. When we look at Aß deposits and neurofibrillary tangles in the higher brain centers of these nondemented patients, we find little if any evidence of inflammation.

If inflammation does cause substantial damage to the Alzheimer's brain, and if many of the inflammatory mechanisms we observe there are similar or identical to those we find in an arthritic joint, you should be able to guess by this point what a potentially useful drug for treating Alzheimer's disease might be. Yes, you're right. We give anti-inflammatory drugs to help arthritis patients; perhaps we should be doing the same for Alzheimer's patients.

There are now, in fact, some 20 published clinical studies suggesting that anti-inflammatory agents slow down or even delay the onset of Alzheimer's disease. Together with Dr. Patrick McGeer of the University of

British Columbia, another pioneer in this field, we found, for example, that elderly arthritis patients presumably taking anti-inflammatory drugs to ease their joints were some five times less likely to exhibit symptoms of Alzheimer's than other patients their age. Dr. John Breitner of Duke University has studied identical twins, only one of whom has Alzheimer's, or one of whom developed Alzheimer's significantly earlier than the other. What distinguishes the twins? Prior history of anti-inflammatory drug use is one of the major things Dr. Breitner has found to be a distinguishing factor. At the Johns Hopkins Medical School, yet another study has evaluated the progress of Alzheimer's disease in some 200 patients for many years. It was found that patients taking anti-inflammatory drugs had a much slower or less severe disease progression than those not taking such drugs.

My laboratory has also conducted a direct clinical trial in which 14 Alzheimer's patients received indomethacin, a common arthritis medication, and 14 other Alzheimer's patients received placebo (a "sugar pill" made up to look just like the indomethacin). No one except my secretary knew which patient was getting which drug, and she kept the code locked in her desk. After six months of treatment, the placebo patients went, on average, downhill by just the amount they were expected to. The indomethacin patients didn't. In fact, they appeared to be slightly better off, on average, than when they started the trial.

Hold on, though. Don't go rushing out to buy some indomethacin. To begin with, this was a very small trial by modern standards. Moreover, even though indomethacin has been around for over two decades, this does not mean that it is completely safe. It is an aspirin-like drug, but some 20 times more powerful. I don't have to tell you what would happen to your stomach if you swallowed 20 aspirin at one time, do I? Indomethacin, like virtually all the conventional arthritis drugs, has side effects, particularly gastrointestinal (stomach) side effects.

Because of these problems, and because anti-inflammatory drugs have not been thoroughly tested in a sufficient number of patients, they are not yet approved by the United States Food and Drug Administration (FDA) as a treatment for Alzheimer's. Perhaps they will be in the near future, however. Currently, the National Institute on Aging is sponsoring a large-scale, multi-center trial of an anti-inflammatory drug in Alzheimer's disease patients. I would not have picked the particular anti-inflammatory drug they chose, but it's a start. If the trial is successful, I suspect that FDA approval will come quickly.

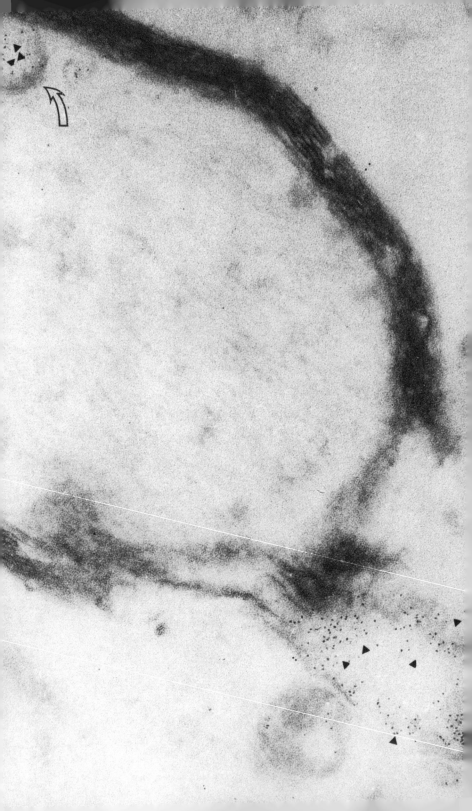

Figure 9

Photomicrograph taken with an electron microscope of a nerve fiber being attacked by inflammatory mechanisms in the Alzheimer's disease brain. The tiny black dots, pointed to in some instances by arrowheads, show the presence of inflammatory molecules that mark the nerve fiber for destruction by scavenger cells or that directly kill the fiber by opening holes in its outer surface. The cell tries to defend itself by extruding (➡) or internalizing (⇨) those parts of its surface that are under attack.

New Directions

HARDLY A WEEK SEEMS TO GO BY without a headline on some new breakthrough in Alzheimer's disease. Indeed, I sometimes worry about this because, like the little boy who cried wolf once too often, I'm afraid the public is going to begin to believe all these miraculous advances mean the problem has more or less been solved. I assure you it hasn't.

In part, many of the headlines reflect the fact that scientists are human. They feel deeply about their research, and when they get a positive result they're usually quite certain of its paramount importance. If their findings are published in *Science* or *Nature* or some other prestigious scientific journal, the research usually gets covered by the news media and publicity results. When interviewed about it, the scientist, being human, will proudly extol the virtues of his or her own work. Other scientists asked to comment are unlikely to be critical in public. About the worst you'll ever hear is something on the order of, "We need more time to follow up this very interesting study."

But often the breakthroughs really are breakthroughs, and everyone agrees. Particularly in the past decade, with the advent of the new molecular genetic techniques, we are finally beginning to understand the root causes of Alzheimer's disease. We have reached consensus over many troubling issues, and Alzheimer's scientists are beginning to pull together as never before. The work on the presenilins, for example, was undertaken as a collaborative effort by scientists at multiple institutions in the United States and Canada—scientists who had always been hot competitors in the past. Likewise, I'm proud to have active joint collaborations with over a dozen investigators around the country.

Let me give you a brief summary of what I consider to be some of the most promising new developments that you'll likely see headlines about in the near future.

To begin with, the diagnosis of Alzheimer's disease itself is being hotly pursued. As noted earlier in the book, physicians understandably don't like making a diagnosis as serious as Alzheimer's without some objective clinical test to back them up. In the past few months, a leading company in Alzheimer's research, Athena Neuroscience, has begun to provide just such a clinical test. Your physician sends them blood and cerebrospinal fluid samples from the patient, Athena does the lab work, and the results are returned to your physician to go along with his or her diagnosis. Again, the test isn't 100 percent accurate, but the findings can lend greater certainty to your physician's conclusions.

The test is based on several recent discoveries, beginning with something we've already talked about: patients who possess apolipoprotein E4, which can be determined from a blood sample, are at increased risk. The Athena diagnostic probes the patient's apolipoprotein E type. Mutations in presenilin 1 are also checked. In addition, amyloid ß peptide (Aß) and certain fragments of neurofibrillary tangles can leak out of the brain and may be picked up in the cerebrospinal fluid, a liquid that flows through the brain and spinal cord. The Athena diagnostic measures Aß and tangle fragments in a cerebrospinal fluid sample from the patient.

The test is somewhat lopsided with respect to accuracy. If it gives a positive result, then it will be correct about 90 percent of the time. In fact, if a presenilin 1 mutation is found, the test will be conclusive virtually 100 percent of the time. Add this to your physician's skill in diagnosing Alzheimer's disease, which can be as high as 95 percent in the right hands, and you've got just the answer you didn't want: the patient almost certainly has Alzheimer's. On the other hand, if the test comes back negative things aren't so clear. You may find out, for instance, that the patient doesn't have apolipoprotein E4 or a presenilin 1 mutation, but that's no guarantee that a patient is free from Alzheimer's. Many patients without apolipoprotein E4 or a presenilin 1 mutation get the disease; having them only increases your susceptibility. Similarly, it may be found that the patient lacks tangle fragments in the cerebrospinal fluid. Again, however, this finding isn't universal for all Alzheimer's victims. A negative test, in fact, picks out patients who are free from Alzheimer's only with about 60 percent accuracy. For these reasons, the Athena test is only recommended as part of a thorough evaluation by your physician and can only be ordered by a physician.

Taking a blood sample isn't really a big deal, as you probably know from having donated blood. Obtaining a sample of the cerebrospinal fluid, however, isn't particularly pleasant and often causes a colossal headache afterwards. Whether you want the increased information provided by the Athena test is, therefore, something you should carefully discuss with your physician.

We may be close to another improvement in Alzheimer's diagnosis based on new work that uses sophisticated X-ray and other scanning techniques. Positron emission tomography, the PET scan, for example, shows the general activity of different brain regions. When there's a problem, the affected region may exhibit reduced activity. A recent study of people who appear mentally normal but who are both apolipoprotein E4 positive and have an immediate relative with Alzheimer's found many who have depressed activity in two brain regions where Alzheimer's patients typically do. Some of these patients have gone on to develop Alzheimer's. Similarly, a series of studies from Oxford University has revealed that we may be able to diagnose Alzheimer's disease and even see it developing by using computed axial tomography, the CAT scan, to survey an area near the inner surface of the temporal lobe. From autopsies, we know that this is a brain region that is very hard hit in the disease. What the Oxford scientists have suggested is that we can see this area in living patients much better if we tilt the CAT scan apparatus slightly, sending the X-rays into the brain at a different angle. When this is done, a consistent thinning of the inner surface of the temporal lobe is observed in Alzheimer's victims compared to normal elderly people. Moreover, with repeated CAT scans of the same Alzheimer's patients, progressive thinning may be seen.

Improved methods of diagnosis, from the Athena test to brain scans, will become increasingly important as new and better drugs come along for Alzheimer's. The early years of the disease can be good years, with an active, full life. I even know one lady who was diagnosed two years ago and still plays bridge far better than I do (although this is not necessarily a high compliment, considering my level of skill). If we can identify patients early through better diagnostic tests, then perhaps we can hold them there with new and better drugs. Moreover, to the extent that diagnostic tests such as PET scans can track changes in the condition of patients, we will have an important new tool for drug development. Presently, we rely on psychological assessments that can vary a lot from patient to patient (and even from day to day in the same patient) in order to determine whether or not a drug is helpful in treating Alzheimer's. An objective biological measure in which we could actually see how a drug was affecting the brain might be a big improvement.

New treatments for Alzheimer's should be coming soon as well, probably in the next year or two, based on drugs that are now undergoing clinical trials. Many of the drugs, like Cognex and Aricept (see the chapter on acetylcholine), work by boosting neurotransmitters, the molecules that carry messages throughout the brain. Unlike Cognex and Aricept, however, some of these pharmaceuticals appear to act on more than one neurotransmitter. This may be an improvement since several neurotransmitters appear to be lost in the course of Alzheimer's, not just one. Alternatively, as noted earlier in the book, there is a widespread loss of the nerve cells that receive the messages carried by neurotransmitters. Boosting the messages may therefore be something akin to beating a dead horse.

Other compounds now in clinical trials have mechanisms of action that are more broadly based than facilitating neurotransmitters. Selegeline, vitamin E, and ginkgo bilboa, for example, have anti-oxidant properties. This may be helpful by reducing the damage done when cells burn oxygen to provide energy (the burning is chemical and therefore flameless, of course). Toxic oxygen byproducts called reactive oxygen and nitrogen species or free radicals build up over time as a result of these processes. This isn't a problem for most cells because they turn over so rapidly. Skin cells, for example, are sloughed off and replaced on a daily basis so that they don't have time to accumulate a lot of oxidative damage. Nerve cells, on the other hand, don't turn over at all. Every nerve cell in your brain has been with you since birth. Given decades, oxidative damage may become significant for nerve tissue, so it's not unreasonable to think that anti-oxidants might help brain cells cope with at least one of the problems they face with advancing age. Toxic oxygen byproducts are also produced in the course of inflammation, which we know is involved in Alzheimer's disease, and has recently been suggested to be a potential risk factor in Alzheimer's.

How effective the anti-oxidants may be in Alzheimer's (or normal brain aging) remains unclear despite exaggerated claims and selective citation in some of the "new age" or "alternative medicine" textbooks you may find at the book store. Always cited and discussed in these books are clinical trials that have been successful, but you usually need to read the original research reports to find out how marginal the positive effects were. Trials where no benefit at all was obtained are almost never mentioned. Investigators at the University of Nebraska Medical School, for example, recently conducted a very thorough study of selegeline and found it to have absolutely no therapeutic effect in Alzheimer's disease. A highly publicized recent study with ginkgo in 309 probable Alzheimer's patients showed approximately a 6 percent improvement on a particular memory test called the Alzheimer's Disease Assessment Scale. Given so small a change, it is perhaps not surprising that the physicians evaluating patients were generally unable to see any difference. Nonetheless, ginkgo is virtually the only health food store remedy where the manufacturer has had the courage and honesty to actually conduct a rigorous trial of its product. The company, Dr. Willmar Schwabe Pharmaceuticals, is to be applauded and, considering ginkgo's apparently mild adverse reaction profile, it should do well. Just consult your physician before you try it on an Alzheimer's patient in your care.

Slightly less far along on the path to new drug discovery is research with glutamate. Glutamate is another neurotransmitter molecule that brain cells use to signal to each other. To get the glutamate message, the recipient cell must possess glutamate receptors, which catch the glutamate molecules as they are passed from one cell to the next. Too much glutamate, however, can overstimulate nerve cells and cause their death. Some scientists are therefore studying mechanisms that normally control glutamate levels in the brain and that might become defective in the Alzheimer's brain. Other investigators, including Dr. John Morrison and his colleagues at Mt. Sinai Medical School, have found age-dependent decreases in a particular form of the glutamate receptor, the NMDA receptor. Such changes could cause problems in just the wrong brain areas for an Alzheimer's patient. The hippocampus, for example, is loaded with glutamate receptors, uses glutamate pathways in memory processes, and is especially vulnerable to Alzheimer's pathology.

Gary Lynch and his collaborators at the University of California, Irvine, and Cortex Pharmaceuticals have been studying yet another receptor involved in glutamate transmission. It's called the AMPA receptor. Ampakines, drugs that stimulate the AMPA receptor, appear to reverse memory deficits in old rats. Perhaps they might do so as well in Alzheimer's patients. Clinical trials to establish the safety of ampakines in humans are now underway.

From having read the earlier chapters, you may well be able to guess some of the other promising approaches that are being taken toward developing new Alzheimer's therapies. Premarin, an agent commonly used for estrogen replacement therapy during and after menopause, is being examined because of the link with declining estrogen levels in elderly women and their increased susceptibility to Alzheimer's disease. Cholesterol-reducing drugs are being considered because they might lower concentrations of apolipoprotein E4. Agents that block the entry of calcium ions into brain cells could prove useful, since too much calcium can kill cells and there is evidence that nerve cells in old animals may let calcium in too readily. Blocking the production or deposition of Aß also seems worth pursuing because the Aß molecule is clearly associated with damage in the Alzheimer's brain. Hormone-like molecules called growth factors are being tried as well, both in Alzheimer's disease and other neurodegenerative disorders such as amyotrophic lateral sclerosis (ALS) (Lou Gehrig's disease). In vitro (in a test tube) the growth factors help cells survive and, in the case of nerve cells, maintain their connections. Perhaps they can help offset the loss of nerve cell connections in Alzheimer's disease, or even encourage new growth.

Our prospects for understanding the fundamental pathologic processes of Alzheimer's disease may have improved recently thanks to another development at Athena Neuroscience, the same company that produced the new diagnostic test discussed earlier in this chapter.[3] The Athena scientists have a line of mice that exhibit amyloid ß peptide (Aß) deposits like those in Alzheimer's disease, and, more recently, a second, similar line has been developed by Dr. Karen Hsiao. The way these animals were produced utilizes virtually the gamut of techniques available in modern biotechnology. First, the gene that codes for Aß was isolated from a family that had hereditary Alzheimer's disease caused by a mutation in their Aß or APP gene. The mutated gene

---

3 • Yes, I also own stock in this company (actually, their parent company, Elan Pharmaceuticals). I often collaborate with Athena's scientists, and I think they do great work. Alternatively, I'm no genius on Wall Street so, once again, caveat emptor!

was then synthesized so that many copies were available. By putting a copy into the egg cells of a female mouse, each egg not only carried the normal complement of mouse genes but also the abnormal human Aß gene. When successively bred, a line of mice that expresses and deposits Aß in their brains was produced. These "transgenic" mice are an important step forward because now we can examine the processes that cause Aß deposition and try ways to prevent it that we could not with living Alzheimer's patients. Unfortunately, neither the Athena mice nor those from Dr. Hsiao exhibit tangle formation, the other cardinal sign of Alzheimer's. Dr. Hsiao's mice appear to develop cognitive impairments, but to my knowledge nothing in this area has been published by Athena for their mice. Lacking these elements, the mice provide a useful model system but only for one part of the problem.

How the mice feel about all this may be a point worth concluding this chapter with, as a small but vocal segment of our population appears to take a very dim view of any use of laboratory animals for research, and the Athena and Hsiao transgenic mouse models, for the first time, makes this a real possibility with respect to Alzheimer's disease.

Like virtually all the scientists I know, I do not take the use of laboratory animals casually. As a matter of fact, I have two beagles at home and I don't much care for the use of this breed for cardiovascular and other research. Still, it is sometimes necessary, and I have to recognize that.

Beagles, of course, inspire much more tender feelings in human beings than mice do. Nonetheless, even the use of mice for research must be carefully justified, and I applaud responsible animal rights organizations for forcing scientists to do just that. Even if we weren't constrained by ethics from doing all but the most essential research on laboratory animals, however, practical considerations would still exert considerable force. The fact is that laboratory animals cost a small fortune to buy and maintain, and the animals themselves are often difficult and sometimes dangerous to work with. I cannot, for example, go near a rat, mouse, rabbit, cat, or hamster without having an asthma attack. Getting rat blood in an open sore on my finger could easily be as lethal to me as it might have been for the rat.

If the Athena mouse or some other model proves useful, it may take a hundred thousand or more of these animals to solve Alzheimer's disease. Balance that against the statistic that there are now at least 10 million Alzheimer's victims in the world. I cannot tell you how to decide. I can say, however, that before anyone condemns the scientists, they should spend a few days as caregiver for a severe Alzheimer's patient. Or give a few hundred lectures to the distraught families who now have a mother, father, sister, or brother who has been reduced to incoherent jabbering by this horrible disorder. It might change the mind of even the most vociferous animal rights activist.

Green Barley Juice, Snake Oil, and other Dubious Remedies

THOUGH I HATE TO SULLY A BOOK ABOUT science, I would be remiss if some discussion weren't offered about various home remedies you've undoubtedly heard of as cures for Alzheimer's disease.

I'll try to make this short: with the possible exceptions of vitamin E and ginkgo, no health food store remedy or nutritional supplement has been shown to cure, halt, or improve Alzheimer's disease. No drug, no mineral, and especially no over-the-counter patent medicine. So why do I continue to get desperate families in my office with a bottle of snake oil in their hands and a hopeful look in their eyes? Who would be so mean as to sell this stuff as a cure? Alzheimer's is bad enough without some unscrupulous characters trying to make a buck out of it. Worse still, they've learned how to turn scientists and their necessarily plodding ways into the villains. That way, anytime an objection is raised to their products' claims, they've got a pat answer: the conspiracy of establishment scientists.

Let's analyze that thought a minute. Here you have a scientist who is making an astonishingly small amount of money compared, for example, to the physicians who will ultimately prescribe the drug the scientist is working on. His only hope for fame, much less fortune, is in discovering the drug and getting it to the market. Do you think he's going to sit on his answer so he can get a few more years time for research in his dreary lab?

Not unless he has Alzheimer's!

The problem for the scientist is that he or she has to provide careful proof to back up any claim. At heart, an investigator may be every bit as unscrupulous as a quack medicine salesman, but he also knows that he'll be pilloried by his colleagues if he doesn't test thoroughly. So he does. He performs basic research to find out what kind of drug is needed for a particular disease. Then he performs more research to find a drug that will do what's needed. Then the drug is tested in laboratory animals, if possible, to determine if it really does what it's supposed to do. Hopefully, without killing the subject. Finally, the scientist must round up a lot of physicians and patients and statisticians, and try out the drug for real.

This takes time. It's an agonizingly long process during which you have a near certainty that many patients will die because they can't get access to your new drug, which is currently undergoing restricted tests. The converse, rushing headlong to market without adequate testing, can be even worse. You remember thalidomide babies, don't you?

As hopeless as Alzheimer's disease may be, and as profitable as it would be to put out some half-baked drug for it, it's simply not ethical to do so. You may argue that Alzheimer's patients will inevitably worsen and die anyway, so why not give them experimental drugs right now, even if you don't yet know the long-term side effects? That's a legitimate position. But what if the experimental drug does cause some horrible deformity, or unexpectedly blinds the patient after a few months of use, or simply kills the patient? Worse, what if, during this time, some other new drug is proven to cure Alzheimer's? You may already have bartered away your chance to use it on a desperate hope.

These are important concerns and difficulties that are faced by legitimate scientists working to cure disease. They aren't there for the sake of the scientists. On the contrary, they get in our way. They are there for the protection of the public. People in health food stores do have a point that medical science often overlooks the obvious. They argue, quite rightly, that good nutrition and freedom from toxic chemicals have not been explored sufficiently as a means to fight disease. But don't tell me these things will cure Alzheimer's unless you've done the hard work of proving it. What few studies that have been done strongly suggest that nutritional factors aren't involved in Alzheimer's. The growing number of unfounded, untested claims that some "natural" product or other will help an Alzheimer's patient simply distracts us from serious work. Of that I can personally attest.

Over the past few years, I've increasingly found myself spending time talking with people about some new home remedy or other they want to try on their relative with Alzheimer's. Here are some examples. Perhaps you'll recognize the players.

One elderly gentleman came in with a tattered list of things he had bought in a health foods store. He wanted to combine them into a cocktail and force-feed it to his brother with Alzheimer's. I can't remember all the ingredients, but green barley juice was one that will probably always stick with me. I asked him if he thought his brother would approve (or would have done so before he got Alzheimer's disease). "Oh no!" the gentleman replied. "My brother was a physician and he hated stuff like this."

More serious are the unscrupulous health foods brokers who ply on half-truths about nutrition, medicine, and biology. I was visited recently by one of their salesmen, a genuinely nice, genuinely well meaning man who lives close by. He told me how his product cured everything from chronic backache to cancer. How it had completely restored an Alzheimer's patient in Idaho. How it had changed his own life. And he meant and believed every word he said, I have no doubt.

I began to look through the product literature he brought with him. Interestingly, there was no claim about backaches or cancer or Alzheimer's. In fact, if you read carefully, there really wasn't a claim about anything except that you could make a lot of money distributing jars of the stuff in what appeared to me to be a pyramiding scheme. Well, naturally, the salesman said testily, our literature doesn't make claims. In fact, we're never allowed to mention such things in meetings with company officials. Look, right here on the label, "a potassium supplement" is all it says.

And that's all it is. The company officials are smart enough to know that they'll get into trouble making any claim other than a loosely regulated one such as mineral supplementation. Why should they make grandiose promises, when they know their salesmen, who genuinely believe in the product, will do so for them.

"Where has the product been tested for all these cures?" I asked the man.

"In the greatest laboratory in the world," he answered, "the human body." He was right, too. The brochure clearly said so on page three. The discoverer and his son carried the title of doctor. Doctor of what, I wondered, and from where? The brochure offered no answer.

Because the man was so sincere, and seemed to care so much about the plight of Alzheimer's patients who had not yet tried his company's remedy, I asked him why the company had never done the necessary trials to establish effectiveness for the disease. Surely if you have such a cure, it's the only humanitarian thing to do, I said. It would also make the manufacturer about a hundred thousand times more money than they were currently receiving.

There was no answer to that one. He said he'd bring it up next time he met with company officials. I won't hold my breath for their response.

As indicated in the previous chapter, I also must confess to a lack of patience with certain "new age" texts on brain aging, particularly those that spend a lot of time talking about the effects of stress on the brain. To begin with, these books typically use the term stress in a very careless way. A number of physiological stressors—for example, oxygen or glucose deprivation—do cause injury to nerve cells. So also do high concentrations of adrenal steroids. However, these are not necessarily the same thing as psychological stressors—the pressure of work, driving through rush hour every day, or a failing marriage. Whether the latter have any deleterious physical effects on the brain sufficient to account for brain aging or Alzheimer's disease is completely unknown.

For many people, meditation or other methods used to reach a more tranquil mental state would certainly improve the quality of life. One of the "new age" books, in fact, is based in large part on treating Alzheimer's disease through transcendental meditation. Perhaps you might get your relative with Alzheimer's to try it. I can just see Uncle Joe squatting in the lotus position mumbling his mantra. A former banker, hugely conservative, getting Uncle Joe to say "ommmmmmmmmm" (or to remember it) would probably be worth a caregiver of the year award. Just don't expect Uncle Joe's Alzheimer's to get any better. It won't.

Still, there isn't a cure or therapy for Alzheimer's disease yet. And who am I to deny that somewhere out there a flower grows that contains the answer, like the penicillin in bread mold. Moreover, many people feel better psychologically doing something, anything, even when they know it's ridiculous, rather than just waiting passively for the inevitable. More power to them. So here, for what its worth, are my golden rules for home therapy and Alzheimer's.

First, ask yourself or the salesman why the company doesn't claim on its label that their product is useful for Alzheimer's.

Second, don't confuse stimulation or other physiological effects with therapy. Caffeine is a stimulant that many people, perhaps wisely, avoid. What they don't know is that other compounds that look and act very much like caffeine abound in many of the so-called "natural" drugs they take. Theophylline, for instance, is found in tea, and is a sister compound to caffeine. Not knowing that they're getting a stimulant, many people will claim to feel better or more energetic (or even rejuvenated) when in fact all they're really getting is a caffeine-like high. Similarly, many plant products commonly found in health food "supplements" contain mild laxatives. Regularity often does wonders for the disposition. But it won't stop Alzheimer's disease.

Third, be aware that human beings are hugely affected by something called the placebo response. That is, you give a group of patients a sugar pill, tell them it's medicine that will help, and sure enough a surprising number will report that it worked. Such cures are the stock in trade of the quack medicine salesman.

Fourth, don't give anything to patients that they themselves wouldn't give to you if your situations were reversed. Just because someone is in your care doesn't mean you have the right to abrogate everything they believed in before they developed Alzheimer's.

Fifth, ask your doctor if it will kill anybody to ingest the stuff you've bought.

And last, don't give any home remedy or health food supplement or patent medicine to a patient unless you're prepared to try it first.

What You Can Do to Fight Alzhiemer's Disease

THERE ARE TWO VERY IMPORTANT THING'S you can do to fight Alzheimer's. The first is obviously to support research now, in the hope that there will be a cure for Alzheimer's before you or your children get it. Hopefully, this book will help you see that an Alzheimer's cure in our lifetime is not so far-fetched an idea. We really are making rapid progress. Thus, as much as it pains me to write that there is virtually no hope for your relative who now has severe Alzheimer's, it gladdens me to believe that Alzheimer's will not be something our children must face. With your support, we will find a cure.

For many years, the bulk of financial support for Alzheimer's research came through the federal government by way of National Institutes of Health grants to scientists. The Alzheimer's Association, one of the finest nonprofit charitable organizations ever created, has also played a substantial role. They've put together local chapters almost everywhere, with support groups for families, newsletters and brochures, and money for research.

As the United States government has tried to come to grips with its overwhelming debt, it's become increasingly difficult for federal funding of Alzheimer's research to keep pace with the exciting new developments that are occurring in the field. Even though Alzheimer's funding has actually fared relatively well compared to some other equally horrible human diseases such as multiple sclerosis and Parkinson's, it's still true that we presently spend about a penny trying to find a cure for Alzheimer's disease for every dollar we spend taking care of Alzheimer's victims. It's not for me to say that our priority should be Alzheimer's research over defense or savings and loan bailouts. We elect politicians, not scientists, to make such judgements. But if we make it our credo that federal spending must be cut, that the government cannot any longer afford to take care of all our needs, no matter how worthy, then we must begin to look within our own communities for the dollars that make Alzheimer's research possible.

You could begin with a contribution to the Alzheimer's Association. They're located at 919 North Michigan Avenue, Suite 1000, Chicago, Illinois 60611, Telephone (800) 272-3900. As noted above, they're a tremendous organization with chapters all over the country. They keep almost nothing for their overhead, sending almost every dollar out to support groups of

Alzheimer's families and scientists like me who do Alzheimer's research. I wish I could say the same about some other organizations that do nation-wide mailings about Alzheimer's. My advice is to look for the Alzheimer's Association name. If it's there, then that's where I'd send my money

If you want to keep your contribution within your community, that's also possible. The Alzheimer's Association has local chapters almost everywhere. Just look for them in the phone book. You might even consider directly supporting a scientist in your area. I have several colleagues who've managed to keep their Alzheimer's programs together this way and my own institution, the Sun Health Research Institute, would not even exist without community support. To find out if there's research being done near where you live, try calling your local Alzheimer's Association chapter. They'll probably have an answer. The second thing you can do to fight Alzheimer's may not be as obvious as donating money to research, but it has the great advantage that it's available to everyone, rich or poor.

Donate your brain to research.

You see, rats, cats, and dogs don't get Alzheimer's disease; just people do. Thus, (with the possible exception of the Athena mouse) we have no experimental model based on laboratory animals in which to study the disease. To understand Alzheimer's and to find a cure, one must look at its victims. That's the only way.

Without tissue from deceased Alzheimer's patients, we have nothing to examine, nothing to run experiments on, nothing to do at all. We'll never find a cure without the brain tissue that brain autopsies provide.

For myself if I had Alzheimer's disease, I can think of nothing better than to go down fighting the disease that killed me. Giving my brain for scientific research, a necessary part of which will be an autopsy diagnosis, will be my finest gift.

You, the non-Alzheimer's victim, also can play an important role in this endeavor. Suppose a scientist finds a critical missing link in your relative's brain that he or she believes is the cause of Alzheimer's. How do you prove it? You must show that the missing link is present in a normal brain (or vice-versa). Without normal brain tissue, scientists are equally dead in the water. We have nothing to compare so as to be able to state that something we found was normal or abnormal.

For these reasons, I urge you to recognize how important a brain autopsy and contribution of tissue is to Alzheimer's research. Then recognize that what's good for the goose is good for the gander. Sign yourself up right after you sign up your loved one. You may end up playing the most important role in the crucial experiment that cures this terrible disease. Convinced? I hope you are. And to make things easy, you'll find on the last page of this chapter a list of people you can contact to sign up at a facility near you. Be sure to tell the first person you speak to that you're interested in participating in their brain autopsy program for Alzheimer's research. I suspect you'll get a warm reception. If you can't locate some place convenient on the list, call the Alzheimer's Association chapter in your area. They may be able to help.

Donating your brain and that of an Alzheimer's victim you may care for or know has a second benefit beyond its crucial role in research, and this is a benefit to your family. You see, when we do an Alzheimer's study, it's obviously essential that we know exactly what we're studying. Before any experiments are done an experienced physician will therefore examine the brain in detail. As you've learned, such an examination is the only sure way to diagnose Alzheimer's. The evaluation will be communicated to your family, and in this way your children won't be left wondering if Uncle Joe really did have Alzheimer's or something else. The worry isn't worse than the disease, but it's not trivial either. Interestingly, it's also necessary to perform a complete evaluation of the brains of normal people like yourself when they've signed into an Alzheimer's research program and come to autopsy. In making scientific comparisons, it's just as important to know that your normal brains are normal as it is to know that your Alzheimer's patients had Alzheimer's. For this reason, if you take my advice and enroll in a brain donation program for Alzheimer's research, you yourself may get a little present—although you won't be around to enjoy it fully. Sometime after you die, your relatives will receive a letter signed by an expert in the evaluation of brains and attesting to something you may have argued for many years with your brothers, sisters, cousins, and friends. The letter will say that, indeed, you had a normal brain.

WHERE TO CALL TO PARTICIPATE IN OR FIND OUT MORE ABOUT ALZHEIMER'S RESEARCH IN YOUR AREA

Stanley H. Appel, M.D.
Alzheimer's Disease
Research Center
Department of Neurology
Baylor College of Medicine
6501 Fannin, NB 302 Plaza
Houston, Texas 77030-3498
OFC: (713) 798-4073
FAX: (713) 798-3854

Leonard Berg, M.D.
Alzheimer's Disease
Research Center
Campus Box 8111
Washington University
Medical School
4488 Forest Park Boulevard
St. Louis, Missouri 63108-2293
OFC: (314) 286-2881
FAX: (314) 286-4763

Paul D. Coleman, Ph.D.
Department of Neurobiology
and Anatomy, Box 603
University of Rochester
Medical Center
601 Elmwood Avenue
Rochester, New York 14642
OFC: (716) 275-2581
FAX: (716) 273-1132

Jeffrey L. Cummings, M.D.
Department of Neurology
and Psychiatry
University of California,
Los Angeles
710 Westwood Plaza
Los Angeles, California
90024-1769
OFC: (310) 824-3166/206-5238
FAX: (310) 206-5287

Kenneth L. Davis, M.D.
Department of Psychiatry
Mount Sinai School of Medicine
Mount Sinai Medical Center
1 Gustave L. Levy Place, Box 1230
New York, New York 10029-6574
OFC: (212) 241-6623
FAX: (212) 369-2344

Steven DeKosky, M.D.
Alzheimer's Disease
Research Center
University of Pittsburgh
Western Psychiatric Institute
and Clinic
3811 O'Hara Street
Pittsburgh, Pennsylvania 15213
OFC: (412) 624-6889
FAX: (412) 624-7814

Dennis A. Evans, M.D.
Department of Medicine
Rush Alzheimer's Disease Center
Rush-Presbyterian Medical Center
1645 West Jackson Blvd, Suite 675
Chicago, Illinois 60612
OFC: (312) 942-3350
FAX: (312) 942-2861

Steven H. Ferris, Ph.D.
New York University Medical Center
550 First Avenue, Room THN312
New York, New York 10016
OFC: (212) 263-5703
FAX: (212) 263-6991

Caleb E. Finch, Ph.D.
Division of Neurogerontology
Ethel Percy Andrus Gerontology Center
University Park, MC-0191
3715 McClintock Avenue
University of Southern California
Los Angeles, California 90089-0191
OFC: (213) 740-1758
FAX: (213) 740-0853

Bernardino Ghetti, M.D.
Department of Pathology,
MS-A142 Indiana University
School of Medicine
635 Barnhill Drive
Indianapolis, Indiana 46202-5120
OFC: (317) 274-7818
FAX: (317) 274-4882

Sid Gilman, M.D.
Department of Neurology
Alzheimer's Disease Research Center
University of Michigan
1914 Taubman Center
Ann Arbor, Michigan 48109-0316
OFC: (313) 936-9070
FAX: (313) 936-8763

John H. Growdon, M.D.
Department of Neurology
Massachusetts
General Hospital ACC 830
15 Parkman Street
Boston, Massachusetts 02114
OFC: (617) 726-1728
FAX: (617) 726-7718

Lindy E. Harrell, M.D., Ph.D.
Department of Neurology
University of Alabama at Birmingham
1720 7th Avenue South, Suite 454
Birmingham, Alabama 35294-0017
OFC: (205) 934-3847
FAX: (205) 975-7365

William J. Jagust, M.D.
Department of Neurology
University of California,
Davis Alzheimer's Disease Center
Alta Bates Medical Center
2001 Dwight Way
Berkeley, California 94704
OFC: (510) 204-4530
FAX: (510) 204-4524

Jeffery Kaye, M.D.
Department of Neurology (L-226)
Oregon Health Sciences University
3181 S.W. Sam Jackson Park Road
Portland, Oregon 97201-3098
OFC: (503) 494-6976
FAX: (503) 494-7499

William C. Koller, M.D., Ph.D.
Department of Neurology
University of Kansas Medical Center
3901 Rainbow Blvd,
Wescoe Pav 1008
Kansas City, Kansas 66160-7314
OFC: (913) 588-6094
FAX: (913) 588-6948

Neil William Kowall, M.D.
Alzheimer's Disease Core Center
Bedford, VAMC
200 Springs Road
Bedford, Massachusetts 01730
OFC: (617) 687-2632
FAX: (617)

William R. Markesbery, M.D.
Sanders-Brown Center on Aging
101 Sanders-Brown Building
University of Kentucky
800 South Lime
Lexington, Kentucky 40536-0230
OFC: (606) 323-6040
FAX: (606) 323-2866

George A. Martin, M.D.
Department of Pathology (SM-30)
University of Washington
1959 N.E. Pacific Avenue
Seattle, Washington 98195
OFC: (206) 543-5088
FAX: (206) 685-8356/543-3644

Marsel Mesulam, M.D.
Alzheimer's Disease Center
Northwestern University
Medical School
320 E. Superior Street,
Searle 11-450
Chicago, Illinois 60611
OFC: (312) 908-9339
FAX: (312) 908-8789

Suzanne S. Mirra, M.D.
Emory Alzheimer's Disease Center
VA Medical Center (151)
1670 Clairmont Road
Decatur, Georgia 30033
OFC: (404) 728-7714
FAX: (404) 728-7771

Ronald Petersen, M.D.
Department of Neurology
Mayo Clinic
200 First Street, S.W.
Rochester, Minnesota 55905
OFC: (507) 284-4006
FAX: (507) 284-2203

Donald L. Price, M.D.
Johns Hopkins School of Medicine
558 Ross Research Building
720 Rutland Avenue
Baltimore, Maryland 21205-2196
OFC: (410) 955-5632
FAX: (410) 955-9777

Joseph Rogers, Ph.D.
Alzheimer's Disease Brain Bank
Sun Health Research Institute
10515 West Santa Fe Drive
P.O. Box 1278
Sun City, Arizona 85372
OFC: (602) 876-5328
FAX: (602) 876-5461

Roger N. Rosenberg, M.D.
Department of Neurology
University of Texas Southwestern
Medical Center at Dallas
5323 Harry Hines Boulevard
Dallas, Texas 75235-9036
OFC: (214) 648-3239
FAX: (214) 648-6824

Allen D. Roses, M.D.
Alzheimer's Disease Research Center
Duke University Medical Center
227 J. and K. Bryan Research
Building Research Drive,
P.O. Box 2900
Durham, North Carolina 27710
OFC: (919) 286-3228
FAX: (919) 684-6514

Michael L. Shelanski, M.D., Ph.D.
Alzheimer's Disease Research Center
Columbia University
Department of Pathology
630 West 168th Street New York,
New York 10032
OFC: (212) 305-3300
FAX: (212) 305-5498

Leon Thal, M.D.
Department of Neuroscience (0624)
University of California
San Diego School of Medicine
9500 Gilman Drive
La Jolla, California 92093-0624
OFC: (619) 552-8585, EXT 3685
(VA) (619) 534-4606
FAX: (619) 534-2985

John Q. Trojanowski, M.D., Ph.D.
Pathology & Laboratory Medicine
University of Pennsylvania
School of Medicine Room A009,
Basement Maloney/HUP
36th & Spruce Streets
Philadelphia, Pennsylvania
19104-4283
OFC: (215) 662-6921
FAX: (215) 349-5909

Peter J. Whitehouse, M.D., Ph.D.
Alzheimer's Disease Research Center
University Hospitals of Cleveland
11100 Euclid Avenue
Cleveland, Ohio 44106
OFC: (216) 844-7360
FAX: (216) 844-7239

READING LIST

There are several publications that may complement this book and warrant your attention. For caregiving, a standard for many years has been *The 36 Hour Day*. It gives down-to-earth advice from expert clinicians as well as from caregivers who have gone through what you are going through now. Absolutely indispensable. Diana McGowen has written a very interesting book, *In the Labyrinth*, based on her experiences trying to get a diagnosis of Alzheimer's disease and living with the early stages of the disorder. The most interesting part is that both the patient in question and the author herself are Ms. McGowen! Not every early Alzheimer's patient may be up to writing an entire book, but there's a valuable lesson here about how much can be done at this stage of the disease. *Hannah's Heirs* by Dr. Daniel Pollen, is also a book I would highly recommend because it blends a readable account of the genetics of Alzheimer's with the story of how hereditary Alzheimer's disease has affected a family.

If you want to try your hand at reading some of the original scientific literature on Alzheimer's research, I urge you to start with Dr. Dennis Selkoe's informative articles in *Scientific American* (volume 265, pages 68-71, 1991 and volume 267, pages 134-142, 1992). More technical still are summaries of the aluminum theory by Dr. Paul Levallois in *Neurology*, (volume 48, pages 1141-1142, 1997), the Aß theory by Dr. John Hardy in *Trends in Neurosciences* (volume 20, pages 154-159, 1997), the neurofibrillary tangle theory by Drs. Heiko and Eva Braak in *Neurobiology of Aging* (volume 16, pages 271-284,1995) or Dr. Michel Goedert in the same volume (pages 325-334), "The Genetics of Alzheimer's Disease," by Dr. Ephrat Levy-Lahad and Dr. Thomas Bird in *Annals of Neurology* (volume 40, pages 829-840), the apolipoprotein E theory by Dr. Allen Roses in *Annals of the New York Academy of Sciences* (volume 802, pages 50-57, 1996), and the inflammation theory written by me, Dr. Patrick McGeer, and our colleagues in *Neurobiology of Aging* (volume 17, pages 681-686). With the exception of Dr. Selkoe's *Scientific American* reviews, these latter articles can probably only be found at a medical school library. Likewise, the even more primary scientific papers they reference will also only be available at a medical school library. Should you have the stomach for them, don't be bashful. Your tax dollars helped pay for the medical school, and you have as much (or more) right to look things up in their library as any scientist.

AFTERWORD

Right now as you read this last page, whether at midnight or early morning, there's a scientist somewhere who's working on Alzheimer's disease. He or she may not have all the answers yet, but if you've gained nothing else by working through this book you know at least that we're trying. Perhaps next year. Perhaps the next. The headlines are coming thick and fast, and I'll try to revise this book every so often to keep you abreast of new developments. A fundamental understanding of Alzheimer's disease and beneficial treatments for it are on their way through research and your support of it. They are the candle that will illuminate the darkness of Alzheimer's disease.

ACKNOWLEDGEMENTS

For their encouragement and criticisms of the manuscript, I'm very much indebted to the following scientists: Dr. Zaven Khachaturian and Dr. Terry Radebaugh of the Ronald and Nancy Reagan Center for Alzheimer's Research; Dr. Mark Emmerling of Parke-Davis Pharmaceuticals; Dr. Patrick McGeer of the University of British Columbia Medical School; Dr. Diane Lorton of the Sun Health Research Institute; and Dr. John Hardy of the Mayo Clinic.

Index

A

acetylcholine (ACh), 63-70, 130
acetylcholinesterase (AchE), 66
aging, 17-23
alcoholism, 33-34
α-secretase, 100-101
aluminum, 71-76
aluminum hydroxide, 76
Alzheimer, Dr. Alois, 1, 15, 39, 42, 53, 55, 99, 102, 108
Alzheimer's Association, 145-147
Alzheimer's disease
  effect on the brain, 39-61
  fighting, 145-150
  occurrence of, 3-5
  patient s experiences with, 31-38
  progression of, 35-36
  risk factors for, 17-30
  what it is, 2-3
  what it is not, 7-15
Alzheimer's Disease Assessment Scale, 70, 132
Alzheimer's Disease Core Center, 153
amino acids, 99-100
AMPA receptor, 133
ampakines, 133
amyloid angiopathy, 10, 12
amyloid β peptide
  about, 99-106
  action in brain, 40-41, 45, 52-57
  apolipoprotein and, 89, 92-93

heredity and, 83-84, 86
inflammation and, 113, 115-116, 118
neurofibrillary tangles and, 110-111
new directions in, 127, 134-135
amyloid precursor protein (APP), 40-41, 100-101, 117
amyotrophic lateral sclerosis, 134
anatomical gift, 147-150
animal research, 135-136
Annals of Neurology, 156
Annals of the New York Academy of Sciences, 156
anti-inflammatory drugs, 119-120
anti-oxidants, 111, 130-131
apolipoprotein E, 24-25, 28-29, 89-97, 117, 127-128, 133
apoptosis, 86
Appel, Dr. Stanley H., 151
Aricept, 68-70, 130
artery hardening, 9-10
arthritis, 7-8, 115, 120-121
asthma, 24, 115
Athena Neuroscience, 96, 126-129, 134-135, 136
atherosclerosis, 10, 13
autopsy importance, 97
autosomal dominant Alzeheimer's disease, 93-96
axons, 43

B

basal ganglia, 48-49
Baylor College of Medicine, 151
Berg, Dr. Leonard, 151
Bird, Dr. Thomas, 156
blood
  -brain barrier, 24
  samples, 126-128
  vessel changes, 10, 28
bovine spongiform encephalopathy,
  11-12
Braak, Dr. Eva, 156
Braak, Dr. Heiko, 156
brain
  Alzheimer's patient, 46-47, 48-49
  donations, 147-150
  normal elderly, 46-47, 48-49
  scans, 128-129
  size of, 21-22, 104
Breitner, Dr. John, 120

C

C1q, 116-117
caffeine, 143
calcium blockers, 133-134
calcium carbonate, 76
cannibalism, 72
cardiovascular disease, 28-29, 91
cell, 80
  membrane, 100
  suicide, 86
cerebellum, 105, 118-119
cerebrospinal fluid sample, 128
Chammoros, 71, 72, 74-75
cholesterol, 28-29, 91
cholesterol-reducing drugs, 133
choline acetyltransferase (ChAT), 63
chromosomes, 80-81
Cognex, 67-70, 130
cognitive skills, 22-23, 103
Coleman, Paul D., 151
Columbia University, 154
complement, 116-117

computed axial tomography (CAT),
  33, 129
Cortex Pharmaceuticals, 133
Cotman, Dr. Carl, 106
Creutzfeldt-Jakob disease, 3, 9, 11-
  12, 33
Cummings, Dr. Jeffrey L., 151
cytokines, 117

D

Davies, Dr. Peter, 63
Davis, Dr. Kenneth L., 151
death, cause of, 5-6
DeKosky, Dr. Steven, 151
dementia, 2, 96-97
dementia puglistica, 24
dendrites, 43
depression, 32-33, 37
Deutsch, Dr. J. Anthony, 64
developments, promising, 125-135
DNA, 11
Down's syndrome, 82-84, 103
Drachman, Dr. David A., 64
Duke University Medical Center, 90,
  93, 120, 153

E

Einstein (Albert) Medical School, 63
Elan Pharmaceuticals, 134
endoplasmic reticulum, 85-86
entorhinal cortex, 48-49, 58-59, 106
epilepsy, 20
estrogen, 26-27
estrogen replacement therapy, 133
Evans, Dr. Dennis A., 152
experimental drug ethics, 138-139

F

Ferris, Steven H., 152
fibrils, 56-57, 102
Finch, Caleb E., 152
Food and Drug Administration, 68, 121
forgetfulness, 35-36

free radicals, 131
frontal cortex, 48-49, 50-51, 52-53

G

Gajdusek, Dr. Carlton, 72
gender, 27-28
genes, 80-81, 90
gene therapy, 93-96
Ghetti, Dr. Bernardino, 152
Gilman, Dr. Sid, 152
gingko bilboa, 130-131, 132, 137
glia, 40-41, 102
glutamate, 132-133
glycolipid, 109-110
Goedert, Dr. Michel, 156
Great Britain, 74
green barley juice, 140
Growdon, Dr. John H., 152
growth factors, 134
Guam, 71, 74
Guamanian dementia, 71
gyri, 47

H

Haldol, 37-38
Hannah's Heirs, 95, 155
Hardy, Dr. John, 84, 156
Harrell, Dr. Lindy E., 152
head injury, 23-24
hereditary factors, 25-27
heredity, 77-87
hippocampus, 48-49, 133
home remedies, 137-144
Hsiao, Dr. Karen, 134-135
Huntington's disease, 95
hydrogen peroxide, 110
hyperphosphorylated tau, 109-111
hypertrophy, 41
Hyslop, Dr. Peter, 84

I

incontinence, 36
Indiana University School of

Medicine, 152
indomethacin, 120-121
inflammation, 24, 113-123, 131
In the Labyrinth 155

J

Jagust, Dr. William J., 152
Johns Hopkins School of Medicine, 120, 153

K

Katzman, Dr. Robert, 43. 104
Kaye, Dr. Jeffery, 152
kidney dialysis, 73-74
Koller, Dr. William C., 152
Kowall, Dr. Neil William, 153
Kuru, 72

L

laxatives, 144
Lee, Dr. Virginia, 43
Levallois, Dr. Paul, 156
Levy-Lahad, Dr. Ephrat, 156
limbic system, 44, 45
liver damage, 68-69
Lou Gehrig's disease, 134
Lynch, Gary, 133

M

McGeer, Dr. Patrick, 119-120, 156
McGowen, Diana, 155
MacLachlan, Dr. Donald, 73
mad cow disease, 11-12
magnetic resonance imaging (MRI), 33
Markesbery, Dr. William R., 153
Martin, Dr. George A., 153
Massachusetts General Hospital, 152
Mayo Clinic, 153
Medicare, 33
membrane attack complex, 118, 122-123

membrane proteins, 85-86
memory, 8, 44, 64
mental function, higher, 44
mental stimulation, 12-14
Mesulam, Dr. Marsel, 153
microglia, 102
Mini-Mental Status Exam, 70
Mira, Dr. Suzanne S., 153
molecules, 80-81
Morrison, Dr. John, 133
motor function, 44
Mount Sinai Medical School, 72, 133, 151
movement disorders, 7-9
multi-infarct dementia, 3, 32
multiple sclerosis, 7, 146
mutation, 18-19
mute, 38

N

National Institute on Aging, 121
National Institutes of Health, 72, 145
natural selection, 18-19
Nature, 125
neocortex, 44, 45
nerve cells, 14, 115, 118, 131
    loss, 1-2, 19-21, 39, 42-43, 83
    repair, 91
neuritic plaques, 1, 10, 15
    amyloid β peptide and, 101-102
    in brain, 39-42, 43, 101-102
    inflammation and, 116
Neurobiology of Aging, 156
neurofibrillary tangle, 1, 15
    about, 107-111
    aluminum and, 72, 73
    apolipoprotein interactions, 92-93
    in brain, 39, 41-42, 52-53, 58-59, 60-61
    heredity and, 83
    inflammation and, 113, 115-116, 119

neurofilaments, 108
Neurology, 156
New York University Medical Center, 152
NMDA receptor, 133
norepinephrine, 65
Northwestern University Medical School, 153
nucleus basalis of Meynert, 64, 65-66
nursing home, 37

O

Oregon Health Sciences University, 152
organic brain syndrome, 5, 34
Oxford University, 129
oxidative damage, 131

P

paired helical filaments, 60-61, 108
paranoid delusions, 37
Parke-Davis Pharmaceuticals, 67-68
Parkinsonian dementia of Guam, 71
Parkinson s disease, 7, 13, 65-66, 146
penicillin, 143
Perl, Dr. Daniel, 72-73
Petersen, Dr. Ronald, 153
phenylalanine, 81
phosphate molecules, 109
physostigmine, 66, 67
placebo response, 144
pneumonia, 5, 38
Pollen, Dr. Daniel, 95, 155
positron emission tomography (PET), 28, 128, 129
potassium supplement, 141
premarin, 133
presenilins, 85-87, 89, 125, 127-128
Price, Dr. Donald L., 153
prions, 10-12
Pruisner, Stanley, 11

pyramidal cells, 42

R

reactive oxygen agents, 110-111,
    131
reading list, 155-156
Reagan, Ronald, 14
reproduction, 18-19
resources, 151-154
risk factors
    aging, 17-23
    apolipoprotein E, 24-25, 28-29
    gender, 27-28
    head injury, 23-24
    hereditary factors, 25-27
    vascular changes, 28-29
RNA, 11
Rogers, Dr. Joseph, 153
Rolaids, 76
Rosenberg, Dr. Roger N., 153
Roses, Dr. Allen, 90, 93, 153, 156
Rush-Presbyterian Medical Center,
    152

S

Scandanavia, 74
scavenger cells, 105-106, 114, 117,
    122-123
Schwabe (Dr. Willmar)
    Pharmaceuticals, 132
Science, 125
Scientific American, 156
scrapie, 11
selegeline, 130-131, 132
Selkoe, Dr. Dennis, 156
senile dementia, 2-3, 15, 24, 34
senile plaque, 1, 10, 15
    amyloid β peptide and, 99-106
    apolipoprotein E and, 89, 92-93
    in brain, 39-42, 45, 52-57
    heredity and, 83-84, 86
    photomicrographs of, 50-53
senility, 2

sepsis, 5, 38
Shelanski, Dr. Michael L., 154
Sisters of Notre Dame, 22-23
skilled care, 36
sloth, 12-13
somatostatin, 65
stressors, 142
Strittmatter, Dr. Warren, 90
substantia innominata, 44, 64
sulci, 47
Sun Health Research Institute, 64, 153
susceptibility gene, 90, 94-95
synapse, 20-21, 43, 63-64

T

tacrine, 67-70
tau, 92-93, 108-110
temporal cortex, 48-49, 129
Terry, Dr. Robert, 43, 104
testing, 33-34, 111, 126-130
testosterone, 26
tetrahydroaminocridine (THA), 67-70
Thal, Dr. Leon, 154
theophylline, 143
36 Hour Day, The, 155
threshold theory, 21-23
tissue repair, 24-25
tombstone tangle, 52-53, 108
toxic shock syndrome, 24
tranquilizers, 37-38
transgenic mice, 134-135
treatments, new, 130-133
Trends in Neurosciences, 156
trisomy 21,
    syndrome 82, 84
Trojanowski, Dr. John, 43, 154
Tums, 76

U

University of Alabama at
    Birmingham, 152
University of British Columbia, 119-
    120

University of California, Berkeley, 152
University of California, Irvine, 133
University of California, Los Angeles,
  151
University of California, San Diego,
  154
University Hospitals of Cleveland, 154
University of Kansas Medical Center,
  152
University of Kentucky, 153
University of Michigan, 152
University of Nebraska Medical
  School, 131-132
University of Pennsylvania, 43, 154
University of Pittsburgh, 151
University of Rochester Medical
  Center, 151
University of Southern California, Los
  Angeles, 152
University of Texas Southwestern
  Medical Center at Dallas, 153

University of Washington, 153

V

Valium, 37-38
VA Medical Center, 153
vascular disorders, 10, 28-29
ventricles, 49
viruses, 10-11, 45
vitamin E, 111, 130-131, 137

W

Washington University Medical
  School, 151
welfare, 37
Wernicke-Korsakoff's syndrome, 33
Whitehouse, Dr. Peter J., 154
Winfrey, Oprah, 14

X

X-rays, 128-129